MULTIPLE
BLES8INGS

MULTIPLE
BLES8INGS

Surviving to Thriving with
Twins and Sextuplets

JON & KATE GOSSELIN
AND BETH CARSON

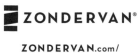

ZONDERVAN®

ZONDERVAN.com/
AUTHORTRACKER
follow your favorite authors

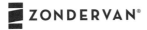 ZONDERVAN®

Multiple Blessings
Copyright © 2008 by Katie Gosselin and Beth Ann Carson

This title is also available as a Zondervan ebook.
Visit www.zondervan.com/ebooks.

This title is also available in a Zondervan audio edition.
Visit www.zondervan.fm.

Requests for information should be addressed to:
Zondervan, *Grand Rapids, Michigan 49530*

Library of Congress Cataloging-in-Publication Data

Gosselin, Jon.
    Multiple blessings : surviving to thriving with twins and sextuplets / Jon and Kate Gosselin
and Beth Carson.
        p. cm.
      ISBN 978-0-310-28902-9 (hardcover, jacketed)
      1. Twins — United States — Pennsylvania. 2. Sextuplets — United States — Pennsylvania.
3. Multiple birth — Popular works. I. Gosselin, Kate II. Carson, Beth. III. Title.
HQ777.35G66 2008
306.874'3092 — dc22   2008016839

Interior photos provided by the Gosselin Family
Interior design by Melissa Elenbaas

Printed in the United States of America

---

08 09 10 11 12 13 14 • 25 24 23 22 21 20 19 18 17 16 15 14 13 12 11 10 9 8 7 6 5 4 3 2 1

To Jon—

Thank you for all you do and for all you put up with. Now I know you meant it when you said in your vows that you would be here "through new and challenging experiences."

You're a wonderful husband, you're an amazing father, and you learned from the best. Your dad—Poppy—would be so proud.

Also to Grandma and Grandpa—

The truest examples of God's unconditional love.

Contents

● ● ● ● ●

Introduction

As I review the pages of this book, Jon's and my story, I still can't believe this is our life! It has taken us these last few years to understand and internalize that this truly is God's plan for us. And when we step back, we realize what an awesome responsibility He has given us. As our youngest children are about to turn four, we still experience challenges daily. But even more, we know that we are so blessed and know that these children, our multiple blessings, and the lessons we have learned through them, are so much more fulfilling than the dreams we could have imagined.

Thank you, Cara, Madelyn, Alexis, Hannah, Aaden, Collin, Leah, and Joel for the privilege of being your parents!

—Kate Gosselin
May 2008

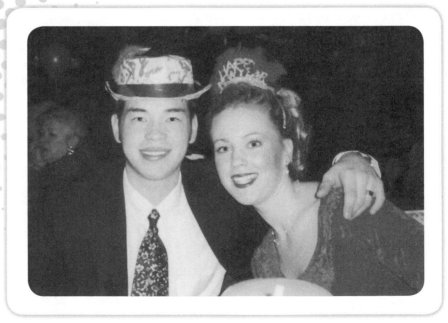

Welcoming 1999, the year we were married.

1 The Calm before the Storm

Trust in the LORD with all your heart
and lean not on your own understanding;
in all your ways acknowledge him,
and he will make your paths straight.

Proverbs 3:5–6

Our first date, if you can call it that, did not go according to plan. Like most little girls, I had dreamed of the day when I would meet my husband, have children, and settle down to live a happily-ever-after kind of life. Unlike most little girls, however, I had an action plan to go with my dream—and it didn't include falling in love with a stranger at a random company picnic. I had been a planner my whole life and took great pride when my plans unfolded exactly as my detailed, scheduled list and calendar said they should.

So when a twenty-year-old soccer player sauntered across a wide green lawn as I sat under a pavilion eating and chatting with friends, I tried not to let my eye get caught on him for long. I was here to be with my friend, not to find a date. But this guy was not aware of my plan and didn't seem to mind having his eye caught on me.

After we danced around each other all afternoon, stealing glances and then quickly turning away, Jon finally walked nonchalantly over to where I stood holding a perfect little sweet-smelling newborn all bundled up in a soft pink blanket. "Are you going to let anyone else have a turn holding that baby?" he asked, holding out his hands toward the bundle in my arms.

That's when I knew I wanted to know more about this cute, friendly, Asian guy who, like me, seemed to melt at the sight of a ten-pound package of sleepy promise. We had that unexplainable good chemistry that seemed to electrify the air around us, and I couldn't help but let my guard down. It seems so silly now, but those first moments of discovery were so fun, so carefree.

I stand in awe when I realize just how much foreshadowing that moment had for the two of us. Who would've guessed at that moment that Jon and I, strangers at the time, would spend endless hours of our lives together handing babies—our babies—from one to the other?

Just six short months after that picnic, Jon, who can never keep a secret for very long, whipped a sparkly diamond ring from his pocket and asked me to be his wife. I was ecstatic and eagerly accepted! But with the very next breath came my list—my long list. See, I may have stepped out of character to fall in love with a stranger in the park, but I was still that little girl with an action plan. I needed a list, in fact, many lists. It complemented my obsessive need to be organized. Type A, take charge, put a label on it, and get the job done—that's me. It wasn't long before I had a to-do list for everyone involved with our wedding: caterer, florist, bridesmaids, and yes, even Jon. I was determined to plan every detail of our beautiful outdoor wedding.

On June 12, 1999, in a friend's fragrant garden in Jon's hometown of Wyomissing, Pennsylvania, Jon and I gathered with a hundred of our closest friends and relatives to begin our life together. Our special day could not have been more perfect: 75 degrees under crystal-clear blue skies. As I look back at pictures of that day, I often wonder what each of us would have done if someone had told us that in less than five years we would be the proud parents of not one, not two, but eight children! Thankfully at that time we were just thrilled and content to go back to our quiet little rented duplex as Mr. and Mrs. Gosselin and dream about our promising and, I might add, well-planned future.

Married life was all I had imagined and more. We were young, healthy, and ambitious, and it wasn't long before baby fever set in. However, though I had always longed to be a mom, the perennial dark question, "What if I can't?" accompanied my dream. That nagging thought would intensify as I soon discovered I had a condition called Polycystic Ovarian Syndrome. Basically that meant I did not ovulate—not a little bit, not ever.

Jon and I were devastated. We worried and prayed, then cried and prayed some more. It seemed like the family we longed for was not going to happen, at least not in the traditional way. I felt empty, betrayed, and broken—like someone had played a cruel joke and stolen all of my dreams when I wasn't looking.

I am not one to wallow in self-pity. I am a doer. Give me an obstacle and I am going to do everything I can to get over it. With a new determination and our eyes on the goal, Jon and I made the difficult decision to seek the expertise of an infertility specialist.

When I thought of infertility specialists, I pictured nice, scholarly

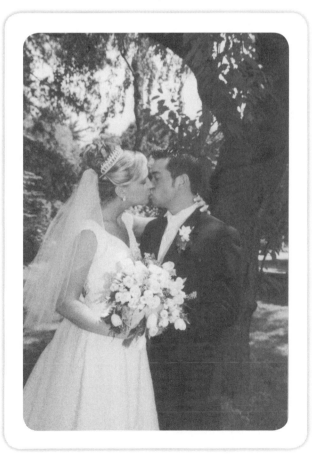

Our wedding day: June 12, 1999.

doctors with all kinds of baby-making potions at their disposal. While I do not want to take any credit away from those wonderful doctors all across this world who have dedicated their lives to seeing dreams of motherhood come true, I must tell you, infertility specialists aren't fun to visit. The process they put you through is painful, risky, and sometimes heartbreaking; however, the miracle they help to bring about is worth every second.

As a Christian I believe Psalm 139:16, which says that all of our days are fashioned for us before we've even lived one of them. In other words, I knew in my heart that God had already ordained exactly if, when, where, and how my baby would eventually come to be — long before I ever stepped foot in that doctor's busy office. I believed this doctor was put in my path simply to carry out what was already my God-given destiny.

It was January of 2000. We had survived the many doomsday predictions that hung over that momentous marker of a new millennium, and now we were anxiously waiting to hear if the painful injections that I had endured for two weeks had worked. The drug, if successful, would cause my ovaries to be stimulated and therefore I would ovulate. I was warned that the risks included producing more than one egg, which could then possibly result in more than one baby.

After our first attempt, Jon and I faced disappointment as I menstruated right on time that month. I felt sad and scared, not to mention I was reeling from the effects of so much hormonal fluctuation, but we decided that we were going to be persistent. We wanted to try again.

Just a few days before the end of my next cycle, I decided to go ahead and take a home pregnancy test. Again. Even though I wasn't late. Somewhere down deep I was hoping that after seeing the neutral white indicator so many times, the odds would work in my favor, and that, one day, by some miracle, that darn little window would be pink. When you are trying to become pregnant, and especially if you have suffered through the wrenching trials of infertility, somehow something as simple as that tiny rectangle on the end of a piece of plastic takes on all the promises of tomorrow's hopes and dreams.

On this particular morning I had woken around 4:30 a.m. to use the bathroom. I did my test, and then, still groggy with sleep, laid it on the bathroom counter and plopped back into my warm bed. It was extremely unusual that I did not camp out in that small, cold bathroom, hovering and pacing, waiting as the minutes ticked by until, as so many times before, I would read the dreaded results. Instead, it was a full hour later when I got up to get ready for work that I remembered to check the test. I couldn't believe my eyes! Could it really be pink? I thought that maybe the glare of the fluorescent lighting was playing tricks on me, so I took the test over to the early morning natural light by the bathroom window. It still looked pink!

Not knowing whether to scream, cry, or pinch myself in case I was dreaming, I ran over and shook Jon. "Jon, Jon! Wake up. Does this look pink to you?" I'm pretty sure a normal man shaken awake by his dear sweet wife who was shoving a urine-christened plastic stick under his nose at 5:30 in the morning and demanding a color analysis would probably have a few choice words to say. Not Jon. He jumped out of bed and threw on the closet light for a closer examination of the now holy stick.

"Look's pink to me, Kate." That's all I needed to hear. I scrambled to get ready for work but kept stopping to look at the beautiful pink. Almost late for work by now, I took off running down the hall waving the stick of my future in the air with one hand and grabbing my car keys with the other. Just as I was about to close the front door, I heard an exuberant "Yesss!" from our bedroom at the end of the hall.

Still not quite believing that the stick was indeed pink, I proceeded to show it to any and all interested nurses at work that day. I reasoned that surely a nursing station full of educated and experienced employees could tell me if one slight pink haze meant something or not. Finally at the end of my shift, I called my doctor who said, "Well, what are you waiting for, Kate? Come get the blood test right now. I'll wait."

"She'll wait," I thought. "How nice."

Waiting took on a whole new meaning as I sat by the phone later at home, hardly breathing. Soon though, the phone rang and with a deep breath and shaky hands I lifted the receiver to my ear. It was positive! I let out a victory scream and then smiled contently, realizing that from that moment on, my life would be forever changed. I was pregnant.

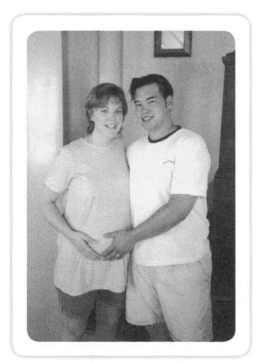

Six months pregnant with twins.
So young, so happy!

2 It Doesn't Get Better Than This

Delight yourself in the LORD
and he will give you the desires of your heart.

Psalm 37:4

Jon and I were filled with awe at the thought of becoming new parents. I was anticipating the fun of decorating the nursery, purchasing all those adorable baby clothes I had admired for months, and learning whether this baby would be a boy or a girl. We happily joked many times that we just absolutely had to have twins; otherwise we would fight over who got to take care of him or her.

To our amazement, our wildest dreams came true. We had been excited to go to our scheduled ultrasound appointment on St. Patrick's Day of 2000, but we were even more excited when we heard those musical words: "There is more than one." We were expecting twins! We had absolutely no inkling of the sleepless nights, endless diaper changes, or even the toothless and drippy grins that would define our next year — nor did we care. We were simply eager to meet these two sweet little gifts that for now were just tiny blips on a fuzzy ultrasound screen.

It was just days later when reality began to set in. I had been out for a leisurely day of shopping with my mother and sister, Chris. We decided to stop for lunch because I had not been feeling well and reasoned that eating something might help me feel better. On the contrary, right then and there at a table in McDonalds began what would be an extremely long stretch of severe "morning sickness." I was in and out of the hospital constantly trying to stave off dehydration.

While I would love to say I tackled this test with the fierceness of a prize boxer in his championship bout, unfortunately that just wasn't the case. I felt that I had paid my dues already in the effort to get pregnant. Did I need to suffer again? This wasn't fair. I didn't want to have to suffer this debilitating nausea that consumed my every waking moment.

I quickly spiraled into a complaining and whining kid, calling my mother every single day to whimper and cry. Eventually, it became necessary for the doctor to prescribe Zofran, which is given to treat severe cases of morning sickness.

Finally, I had relief. I felt as if I had crawled across the desert on my belly and come upon a beautiful and bountiful buffet. It was open season on food—my food, Jon's food, my coworkers' food. It didn't much matter. I was ravenous!

The time spent on my knees with a bucket, however, was soon replaced with bed rest in the hot August weather. The extreme boredom was difficult for me, as I was not accustomed to being stationary for very long ever before in my adult life. Jon rose to the occasion admirably, constantly trying to lift my spirits, going to work, and taking care of all the everyday mundane tasks of keeping a home—such as cleaning, laundry, meals, groceries, and bill paying. It was very comforting to know that we had grown into a couple who, instead of allowing hardships to cause division, chose to rally and draw even closer to each other.

Looking back at that time, we both realize my discomfort was merely God's way of allowing us a small trial run to prepare for the difficulties we were to face in only a few short years.

Finally, on October 8, 2000, all of the dreaded shots, uncomfortable tests, suspenseful ultrasounds, required hospital stays, and endless hours of bed rest would be graciously and faithfully rewarded in the arrival of two bright-eyed, dark-haired beauties. Our daughter, Cara Nicole Gosselin, arrived weighing in at a respectable 5 lbs. 3 oz., followed minutes later by her younger sister, Madelyn Kate, who weighed 5 lbs. 1 oz. Considering that the girls were born just shy of thirty-six weeks' gestation, they were amazingly healthy and required only a short four-day stay in the Neonatal Intensive Care Unit of the Reading Hospital to ensure they were stable and gaining weight. Looking at their delicate, sleepy faces, I could never imagine life being more fulfilling than at that very moment.

Once home with our soft pink-clad bundles, Jon and I concentrated on making a joy-filled happy life for our new family of four. I went back to work as a nurse at the Pennsylvania Dialysis Clinic during the day, and Jon worked the night shift at a local company. This arrangement allowed one of us to be home at all times with our girls. They were growing so quickly — changing it seemed before our very eyes. Mady was not very interested in nursing, so she became a daddy's girl while Cara was quite content to be right by my side.

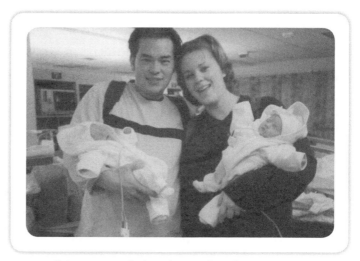

Bringing our babies home, October 12, 2000.

Once again as I reminisce, it strikes me now as very impressive how my husband, at twenty-three years old, was capable of feeding, bathing, swaddling, diapering, dressing, and entertaining two infants all day long and then going to work all night. I also marvel at the grace of a good God who, in His own patient way, was preparing us even then for something that would later test our strength, endurance, tenacity, and sanity — as well as our commitment to each other and to God.

That first year with our two precious babies passed in a whirl of discovery, from their own chubby fingers and toes to stimulating adventures on our almost daily outings. They were now teetering on the brink of toddlerhood, and we felt the inadequacies of our undersized rented apartment becoming more and more apparent.

Consequently, on September 8, 2001, we were fortunate to purchase a tidy three-bedroom home with a one-car garage and a sprawling backyard that just begged for a swing set. It sat on a tranquil tree-lined street with paved sidewalks for tricycles and plenty of garden space in which to plant some spring flowers. We were quite pleased and proud of ourselves for achieving this milestone of owning our own home while we were still twenty-four and twenty-six years old. The responsibility didn't come without its sacrifices, yet that seemed insignificant as we witnessed our young family begin to blossom and thrive.

I had everything I had ever hoped and prayed for: a loving and devoted husband, two chubby-cheeked, silky-haired, pint-sized daughters, a cozy home, and a rewarding career. It was the American dream—but I was having dreams of another sort.

Around the time I set out to plan the girls' first birthday party, I began to daydream about the possibility of having just one more baby. It started as just a quiet whisper in the depths of my soul that soon exploded into a full-fledged heart's cry and desire. I was secretly a bit sad as my two girls sat squishing a slice of their first birthday cake, giggling as we hurried to take pictures to remember their big day. I felt it would be wonderful to give Mady and Cara the gift of being big sisters.

Jon could not have felt more differently. Perhaps he remembered more clearly all the bumps along that long road to parenthood. He would not and could not even bring himself to discuss the possibility. It was an irrefutable, inarguable, and indisputable no! I was so torn between wanting to respect my husband's wishes—after all he was truly concerned about my health—and the undeniable yearning to once again feel the joy of that first faint flutter of a blossoming life within me. I hid the agonizing ache of my broken heart behind the copious daily tasks of caring for the girls and the demands of a sometimes emotionally draining career.

By this time I had realized my goal of working as a labor and delivery nurse. I loved the interaction with each mother as I readied her for one of the most memorable events of her life. I learned early on, however, that to serve my patients most effectively and to guard my own heart, I had to restrain from becoming too emotionally involved. This balance between compassion and professionalism is a challenge to all caregivers.

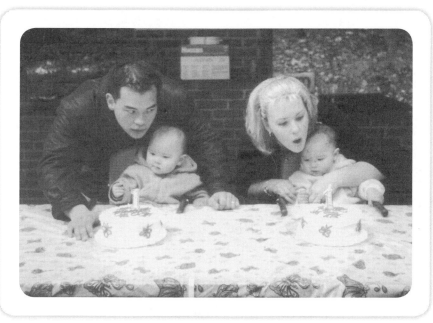

Mady and Cara's first birthday celebration.

Pregnancy could trigger the most exciting or the most despairing time in a woman's life. This fact was not lost on me as I was assigned a teenage girl who was laboring to deliver her first baby. Her anxious mother and stepfather nervously wrung their hands while they alternated between pacing the hallways and smoothing the bed's blankets as their baby girl struggled both mentally and physically with the undeniable reality that she would soon be a mother herself.

This dear, sweet, soft-spoken, and frightened young girl had only the night before revealed to her mother that she was indeed pregnant. Although she was repeatedly asked about everyone's growing suspicions, she had somehow managed to conceal the change in her slight frame with overly baggy clothing, and therefore fuel the fires of denial that had sustained her mother for months.

But now as the family struggled to come to terms with their cold harsh reality, I felt myself softening toward this blonde girl, who yesterday had attended classes as a senior at her high school, listening to the weekend plans of her carefree girlfriends and silently stuffing yet another memo about graduation into her backpack. Jamie talked openly and honestly as I checked her vitals, monitored her contractions, and reassured her that she needed to focus now on the task at hand.

Her distraught mother disclosed that in addition to all of the obvious shocking revelations of the day, was the disturbing fact that the family would never accept a baby fathered by a black man. I knew this fact embarrassed her not because she personally struggled with the race of her grandchild, but because of the bigotry that ran deep in her lineage. She visibly grappled with hurt, anger, concern, confusion, frustration—vacillating between undaunting love for her daughter and dread of what the future might hold. Seemingly grasping at straws during this process, she even alluded that maybe I would be the perfect person to adopt their unexpected, unplanned-for baby.

As the hours of my shift crept by, Jamie continued to labor and I began to feel the achy, stuffy symptoms of a nasty cold. I tried hard to ignore my throbbing head and utter exhaustion, but I soon determined I would need to leave Jamie and hopefully catch up on all of the details of the birth the next day. She and I had bonded, and it is always difficult on both the patient as well as her nurse when a shift change happens as birth is approaching.

I felt reservation as I left that hospital. I just couldn't get Jamie out of my mind that night as I tossed and turned, longing to sleep off my cold but too preoccupied with the details of this teenage girl to allow sleep to come. Her mother's words suggesting that maybe I could adopt their baby rang in my ears as if I had just won the lottery.

Early the next morning I dialed Jamie's room in the hospital to hear if the baby had arrived during the night. Sure enough, he had. I was told he was a handsome peaceful little guy, completely oblivious to the turmoil surrounding his brand new life. His grandma quickly took the receiver, boldly stating that she absolutely needed to speak to me, and she wanted me to please come into the hospital immediately if possible.

She hadn't even finished her plea, and I already knew why she spoke with such urgency. She had mentioned on the phone that she felt that I had been assigned to her daughter for a purpose. I knew in the depths of my being that she was thinking that purpose was to become the adoptive mother of her illegitimate biracial grandson. I felt her heartbeat through the phone as she wrestled with emotions so raw that they threatened to overcome her.

I told her Jon and I would both be there as I myself wrestled with my own mixed bag of emotions. I wondered if this was God's plan, if He was allowing the heartbreak of this unfortunate family to answer my prayers of becoming a mother again. I was shaking with excitement but too terrified to think as we made the short drive to the hospital. We had taken the girls with us, vaguely giving a simple explanation of visiting Mommy's work and getting to see a baby boy who was just born.

When I arrived on the labor and delivery floor, my entire family in tow, to visit a stranger and admire her son, I felt the eyes of the whole ward on me. It was an unspoken "law" that a nurse not allow herself the luxury of becoming attached to her patients. Suspicion lurked as we entered Jamie's room.

We enjoyed a short but intimate visit as we took turns holding the swaddled and drowsy newborn. I quickly learned that Jamie's mother had done her research on adoption and was gently nudging me with facts and information. On the other hand, I was also observing that a certain level of bonding between the family and the baby had already begun. I just kept whispering a prayer for peace. I needed to know without a shadow of a doubt that I was not jumping ahead of God in my quest to quench my thirst for another baby.

We decided the family would visit us at our home the next day. Everything was moving so fast. We needed to tread carefully and be sure this was a decision made out of love and not just desperation — on both Jamie's part and mine.

Throughout the night we weighed the pros and cons. Pros — the baby would have two big sisters to spoil him, I would not have to suffer through possibly another difficult pregnancy, and we would be giving this little boy a comfortable, godly upbringing where he would always feel wanted and valued. Cons — we hadn't thought through this situation for even a full twenty-four hours. What if, even after adopting this baby, I still felt a longing to birth my own child? Would Mady and Cara adjust to this abrupt life-changing decision?

And then there was family. I learned later in the day that our families were less than thrilled with the possibility of us choosing this unexpected detour in our future. While not outwardly discouraging it, my mother acted as spokesperson as she encouraged us to not take one step forward with this adoption until we received a clear, concise, peace-in-our heart response from God. Jon's mother, speaking with unabashed honesty, was a bit more resistant. She adored our girls, cherishing their angelic faces and hair like shiny black corn silk. They were her blood, and by all outward appearances, that was more than obvious. Jon and I were concerned that any baby who was not our own would be forever separate, set aside, different. I was not sure if we, in this case, would be acting in the child's best interest.

Confusion reigned as the four of us sat down that evening for dinner. We had spent the entire day contemplating and praying. As I served the girls their meal, Jon spoke. I don't remember his exact words, but it was as if there was no one else in the room. He was speaking with wisdom and truthfulness, love and strength. I had closed my mouth and just stood listening, which, I must confess, is generally rare for me. Quiet had descended and there it was—that deep-down peace I had been seeking all day.

Seconds later, I felt like I was standing at the edge of the incoming ocean watching the tide tug at my feet on its return pull out to sea. I finally found my voice and whispered, "The answer is no, isn't it?"

Jon replied, "Yes, I think so."

I bent down, serving spoon still in hand and hugged him tightly for a long time.

I was extremely tense and overwhelmingly sad when Jon and I phoned Jamie and her family the next morning to explain our difficult decision. We had thrown them a life preserver and now we were pulling it in before they had a chance to grab it. I understood their hurt, confusion, and even anger.

Just one day before, as the sun was setting, a whole new realm of promising possibilities lay on the horizon, and yet today as the morning mist rose, it revealed a frightening truth. Baby Jeremiah, as he was later named, would be taken home to the house where his mother would put away her childhood memoirs to make room for a crib and changing table. He would have a doting grandmother who would rise to the occasion, fending off any negativity from the outside world. Jon and I would hang up the phone to contemplate what to do with the gaping hole in our hearts that now existed.

Sometimes knowing a decision is the right one to make doesn't make the sting of the consequences any easier to bear. In an attempt to remember our short glimpse into what we prayed would become a long and blessed life for a little boy who touched our lives, Jon and I planted a vibrant flowering hydrangea bush that Memorial Day weekend—our Jeremiah bush. I cried for weeks as I watched the delicate petals turn their brilliant shades of blue, reminded anew of the tender blue-wrapped gift I had willingly relinquished.

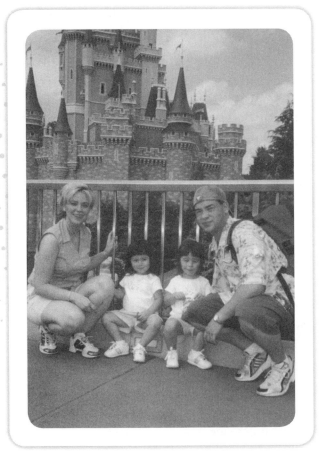

Our very memorable trip to Disney.
Our first and last vacation as a family of four!

3 Our Decision, Our Destiny

Behold, children are a heritage from the LORD,
   The fruit of the womb is a reward.
Like arrows in the hand of a warrior,
   So are the children of one's youth.
Happy is the man who has his quiver full of them.
   Psalm 127:3–5 NKJV

As the days grew warmer, I still mourned the loss of my soured dreams. Once again I turned to my husband with hopes of renewing our well-rehearsed debate on having more children. Jon was worried. He was worried about me, the turbulent months of my pregnancy with the twins, and the potential toll another pregnancy could take on our content and stable family. He hated the thought of more shots, more stress, and more doctor visits. Above all else, Jon worried about the possibility of having twins again.

However, I sensed a crack in his armor. He was softening. He knew only one thing in this world would fill the aching void I felt, and that one thing was downy soft, sweet smelling (most of the time), and had the power to light up the whole room with one toothless grin.

Finally, he agreed to go through it all again—just one more time for three more cycles, a total time commitment of six months. I screeched, dove for the phone, and made an appointment with an infertility specialist right in Wyomissing, just minutes from our home. With my first pregnancy, I had driven an hour away to Allentown, Pennsylvania. Although I obviously had success with that doctor, I felt the convenience of seeing a respected doctor in our own town made much sense, especially with two busy two-year-olds at home.

My first cycle was all that I had remembered—painful injections to help me ovulate, consequent hormonal upheaval, frequent doctor visits, and finally, ultrasounds. I kept my eye on the goal, withstanding it all in the hopes of once again being blessed with the good fortune of holding the much-awaited prize.

To take my mind off some of this all-consuming process, I decided that it would be the ideal time to treat Mady and Cara, who were soon to turn three, to every little girl's dream: Disney World. As with every project I take on, I became obsessed with our family vacation being one of those memories to last a lifetime. With great gusto, I researched every single thing that Disney offered, from sharing breakfast with Cinderella in her exquisite castle to the best time of day to go on the Dumbo ride. Our trip would culminate with a relaxing visit to Jon's aunt and uncle's quaint and quiet cottage for a much-needed detox period from a certain merry mouse and all his inherent chaos.

Jon couldn't grasp my urgency in taking a vacation during such a potentially volatile time on our journey to get pregnant. I, on the other hand, had high hopes of our lives becoming considerably busier in the upcoming year. I felt as if I desperately needed to give this important gift to our curious giggly girls, because, after all, it could be years before we might have the chance to take such a vacation after another baby arrived.

We found out a short time before we left for Florida that my first cycle of treatment was not successful; consequently, I spent one of the best vacations of my life reeling from the rapid surge and then immediate dip in hormones. Nevertheless, although disappointed, I couldn't wipe the giddy smile off my face as I watched our two joyful balls of energy squeal with sheer bliss as we rode the monorail into the park and shook Mickey's white-gloved hand.

We later sat on the white sand beaches bordering our relatives' home contentedly reading, watching Mady and Cara dig in the shimmering warm sand, and soaking up the much-needed quiet. Even now on my worst days, when anarchy rules, I get teary-eyed remembering the simplicity and easygoing pleasures of that smooth and peaceful and truly once-in-a-lifetime vacation.

September was our month of rest in between infertility treatments. It is a necessary reprieve which the body, and I believe the mind also, requires to regain some degree of internal balance before once again enduring the onslaught of hope-filled injections.

Before we knew it, October arrived, bringing with it cool crisp days and the brilliant shades of autumn. I felt an odd calmness descend in my spirit as I watched the girls romping and laughing in the newly fallen crunchy leaves of the backyard. I knew with everything in me that this was the month. This would be the month that we would finally get some positive news.

I couldn't shake the memory either of my dear, sweet, and oh-so-intuitive Mady who, at just shy of three years old, had made a declaration to me with all the soothing surety of a Sunday morning preacher. I had been resting on the couch a short time before leaving for vacation, crying and lamenting over the news that our initial efforts had been in vain.

She came upstairs from her playroom and asked me, "Mommy, why are you crying? Is it about a baby sister or brother?" That wasn't so unusual because, even at their tender young age, I'm sure both Mady and Cara had picked up on the fact that both Mommy and Daddy had discussions involving babies quite often. But then she gently and lovingly caressed my leg with her cottony smooth toddler hand and crooned, "It'll be soon. It'll be soon."

Chills literally scurried up to the top of my head. It was as if God had sent a mighty angel in pint-sized pajamas to whisper reassurance when I needed it the most. I grasped that encouragement, tucked it deep in my heart, and stood on it firmly with all the confidence of an Olympic diver on the highest and scariest platform, about to take the plunge.

Just weeks later, Jon and I sat in a cheerfully decorated office anxiously awaiting the results of my latest set of injections. To our immense relief, our doctor happily reported that by all indications, it was a great cycle. We spent a few moments going over our next steps in the process, which initially would be an ultrasound to determine exactly how many mature follicles had developed.

As at every single meeting, Jon and I expressed on the one hand our serious reservations about the possibility of multiples, and on the other hand our desire for the doctor to fully understand our unwavering position on selective reduction. Selective reduction, in my opinion, is the politically correct term for the process by which a fetus is injected with a lethal dose of potassium chloride, which mercilessly silences forever the rhythmic beats of its tiny heart. Jon and I believe that every life, whether seconds old after conception or a full forty-week term, robustly healthy or horribly sick, fully developed or severely challenged — every life is designed and ordained from God. We would therefore never consider choosing to end that life in any way at any time. Period.

At the scheduled ultrasound on a sunny Sunday morning, the doctor was thrilled. He discovered three mature follicles and possibly even a fourth follicle with the potential to still mature. While Jon and I had that night-before-Christmas kind of anticipation, we were still concerned that all four follicles would somehow be fertilized. Up until that point, when we spoke of multiples, we basically had been referring to the possibility of twins. That was what we had experienced, and so that was our reality. Never did we ever really allow our minds to fully wrap around the idea of multiples turning into more than twins. As if reading our thoughts, our doctor was quick to reassure us that statistically it would be very unlikely that all four or even three of the follicles would be fertilized. He also was completely thorough in giving us an escape route if we so chose. We could simply discontinue the injections and repeat the process in two months, aiming for enough but not too many follicles.

During the car ride home, I silently revisited the deep conversations Jon and I had had before ever setting foot in that doctor's office. We had analyzed the what-if's: What if it was twins? Well, we thought, we did it once; it was certainly doable again. It would mean our family would be definitely complete, doubly blessed. I put a check on the yes side of my mental list.

What if it was triplets? Hmmm. That got a bit tougher. However, as we thought over practical things, like enough room in the house and finances, we decided that although it would certainly be more than we planned, we wanted children, loved children, and would willingly and gratefully accept whatever God handed us. So after a thorough heart search, check again.

That brought us to quads. We tentatively tiptoed into this territory, as if by being quiet enough, we might avoid waking the sleeping giant. Was it really worth dissecting every aspect of this unlikely "giant" if the reality was that we had almost a better chance of being struck by lightning?

Millions of thoughts kept running through my mind, but both Jon and I had an underlying peace even at that early point. We were united in our decision to proceed with that cycle. Even as we walked to the car following the appointment that day, I will never forget Jon's words as he turned to me with complete conviction and said, "We will never regret having too many children. Let's do it!" I let out a deep sigh and felt peace wash over me.

Little did I know at the time that we would be treading on holy ground, and I would need the peace of God to sustain my very life as He walked me through the minefield of surprises that lay ahead. We had carefully weighed all our odds and fearfully yet happily decided to step out in faith and take advantage of my great cycle.

I was given the one final injection of human chorionic gonadotropin, commonly referred to simply as HCG, which was soon followed by the momentous culmination of the whole long involved process: the intrauterine insemination.

No romantic dinner, long-stemmed roses, smooth wine, or flickering candlelight preceded this event. Instead it was a date with a cold sterile room, bright overhead lights, and awkward stirrups. It didn't matter. Nothing could dampen our spirits because we knew that science and humans had given their best efforts, and now the results ultimately lay in God's hands. It was as if we had just run a grueling relay race, the baton had been passed, and the finish line was finally in our sight. As I lay there looking at the ceiling, I prayed, "Please, Lord, let me get pregnant."

A little less than two weeks passed, and on Friday, November 8, I stood at work in a bustling operating room during a routine cesarean section. I had arrived at the hospital a few hours earlier, once again brandishing a white test stick that undeniably displayed the faintest blush of early pregnancy.

My heart was of course skipping in gratitude, but my body felt weak, bloated, and uncomfortable. In a lot of pain and feeling worse by the hour, I actually feared I might collapse at one point during the short surgery while I tried to stay focused on my patient and her newborn baby. Working around women in all stages of discomfort, and some who are enduring flat-out agony, somehow diminishes timid complaints of a bloated and painful belly. I managed to finish my shift and gratefully collapsed into my waiting bed when I returned home.

During a fitful night, I grew increasingly uncomfortable, and as the dark hours crawled by, the pain became a hot scream tearing at my abdomen. I awoke the next morning gasping in pain with a worried Jon begging me to please go to the hospital. Neither one of us at that point even vaguely considered that this pain could possibly be related in any way to the fertility treatments I had received just a few weeks beforehand. Even if it had occurred to us, a hospital visit was most definitely not in my plans that day. My youngest sister, Rissa, was getting married. This was Saturday, her special day, and I did not want to miss it.

I stoically but stupidly gritted my teeth and bore it, though I sat ashen-faced and quiet throughout the entire celebration. My family of course plainly saw that I was in significant discomfort and, after much convincing, I finally agreed to leave the festivities early and was at home tucked into bed by 9:30 p.m.

My hopes of sleeping were completely abandoned by midnight. I was manic with pain. My belly was by that time huge and puffy, and excruciating agony consumed me. I desperately agreed it was time to go the hospital as Jon called his father to come stay with the girls.

I was helped onto a gurney at the hospital, but unfortunately, due to an onslaught of incoming patients, I waited endlessly in the hallway. My stomach looked and felt as if it might explode. Jon frantically tried to explain to the attending doctor that my normally flat belly was now grotesquely distended. Consequently, after enduring an exhaustive exam, I was told a general surgeon would be called into the hospital for consultation, and it was likely they would be prepping me for exploratory surgery very shortly.

As I drifted in and out of consciousness, comforted little by a dose of morphine, Jon was left to answer rapid-fire questions in the doctor's quest to alleviate the source of my agony. Finally it was decided that I should first have an ultrasound done, and all I remember is hearing the OB/GYN resident whisper repeatedly, "Oh my ... oh my ..." Even in my delirious haze, I could tell from the look on the faces surrounding me that something was wrong, very wrong.

The doctor eventually explained that my stomach was completely filled with fluid due to overstimulated ovaries. My ovaries had actually blown up to approximately the size of an average newborn's head! The extreme pain was due to my ovaries rubbing against my other now crowded organs. This condition is only evident in approximately 2 percent of women undergoing similar infertility treatment.

Great, I thought sarcastically, I managed to beat the odds. Miserably weak and sick, I was grateful for the numbing effects of the drugs as the doctor performed paracentesis, a procedure resembling an amniocentesis, which quickly yielded two and a half liters of fluid from my abdomen. Severely exhausted and dehydrated, I spent the next several days in bed recovering from my traumatic experience, first in the hospital and later at home.

On Sunday, while still at the hospital, the doctors, knowing I had had a positive pregnancy test, routinely checked my HCG level. Normally a woman will receive a positive pregnancy result when her HCG level is 25 or higher. That number is then expected to double approximately every thirty hours until about eight weeks after the last menstrual cycle, when it finally levels off. My HCG level was at 200, and it was still one day before I should have gotten my period. By Tuesday, just one day late, that number jumped to 900.

Considering that the normal range is extremely large, no one had mentioned yet that I could possibly be carrying more than one baby. I, however, just knew. I had carried twins before. That in itself did not make me an expert. It was something deeper. Call it mother's intuition or the voice of God. Whatever it was, I just knew that my body, mind, and soul buzzed with the anticipation of something major about to take place.

Jon, on the other hand, ever the optimist, said, "I think it's only one, Kate. Don't jump to any conclusions this early."

●

On the Friday before Thanksgiving of 2003, I saw my infertility specialist and was reminded as I walked through the front doors how science can only do so much; the rest lies in the sovereign plans of an almighty God. That thought rang in my head as the smooth wand of the ultrasound device once again rolled over my uterus. I blinked hard and then stared at the bright screen positioned slightly to my right. Instantly my mind scanned the information. I was a nurse. I had had twins. I had also experienced what seemed like hundreds of ultrasounds. There was no mistaking what I saw, yet instantly I was in a state of denial. I simply could not allow my brain to process what my eyes were telling it.

As if in a trance, we all just continued to stare, as slowly and steadily my doctor began his fateful count. One. Two. Three. Four. I started sobbing. I saw the concentration in the deep dark eyes of my African doctor as he himself tried to remain calm as the images unfolded. I turned to Jon, willing him to say it was not what it seemed. The chill of reality washed over me as I watched my husband — my best friend, cheerleader, and storehouse of strength — slowly drop to his knees at the count of five. Fear stricken and nauseous, he couldn't bear to look anymore. I really don't think anybody wanted to look anymore, but the count continued. Six. Seven. Letter G. Yes, the life-changing fuzzy little blips were being named. They were now A, B, C, D, E, F, and G.

There was a slight upward lilt in the inflection of the doctor's voice as he tried to sound positive. I think as much for his own comfort as for mine, he went on to explain that he was able to detect a fetus in "just" four of the embryonic sacs. As Jon and I tried to catch our breath, a nurse with twenty-five years' experience turned to me and with quiet truth gently said, "Kate, in all these years, I have never seen this many sacs on an ultrasound."

At that moment I felt like lunging at her, holding my hand over her mouth, and shrieking "Take it back" like I did when I was just a kid having a fight with my brother. I didn't, of course, and couldn't because I knew her words were like a bad tasting medicine given to me for my own good. I needed to sit up and think about this harsh dose of truth.

We sat in a stunned silence, which was abruptly broken as the doctor calmly stated, "Kate, when you're done here, come into my office, and we will talk about selective reduction." As if I had been snapped with a rubber band, I grabbed the sides of the exam table and shot up onto my elbows and yelled, "We will never do that!" I felt my first fierce surge of motherly protection over my unborn babies—whether there were two, four, or even seven of them.

I was completely numb as I got dressed. I had an almost unbearable urge to lace up my sneakers and run. I just wanted to feel my heart pumping and the wind in my face as I left behind the black hole of threatening pandemonium that was spreading like a disastrous oil spill. But then it struck me, the problem would come with me. Wherever I went and whatever I did from this day forward, I knew that potentially seven innocent lives were relying on me.

With that thought and maybe a million others scurrying in my mind, I resolutely sat in the sturdy cherry wood chair of the doctor's office. He and I went head to head as he offered facts and information, statistics and grim details of how my life would be at risk. I would never be able to withstand the physical toll that this pregnancy would take. I could die. What about my two sweet little girls at home? They needed me and deserved to grow up having their mommy. The risks for my seven babies also were huge and could not be denied. Assuming that the medical field was capable of getting them to a viable gestational age, usually at least twenty-four weeks, they still stood the risk of suffering premature lungs, blindness, cerebral palsy, and mental retardation—just to name a few possibilities.

I was not swayed. Staring into Jon's eyes with determination, I asked him if he would really be able to stand before the Lord one day and admit that we had allowed our precious babies to be killed in order to make our lives easier and more convenient.

The same concerned nurse who had lovingly stood by my side during the ultrasound begged me to please stop using the word "kill." I didn't. I couldn't. To me that's exactly what it was. Tell me how I as a mother would go about "selecting" which beating heart to snuff out as if it were just a candle. Please don't think I am judging all of the women who are faced with this horrible decision. I can only answer for myself, and "as for me and my house, we will serve the Lord."

Jon, even at the risk of losing me and raising Mady and Cara on his own, unconditionally agreed with me. Who would live and who would die was not a decision that rested in our human hands.

My doctor, visibly shaken, stood and pounded his fists on his desk for emphasis. He declared that it would be a long, arduous, uphill battle that he was strongly urging me not to fight. I realized that I had become a fertility doctor's worst nightmare, and dawn was a long way off.

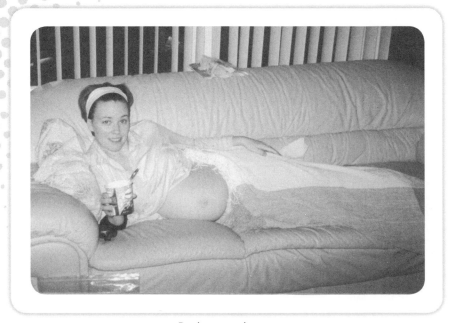

Bed rest at home.

4 What Do We Do Now?

So do not fear, for I am with you;
　　do not be dismayed, for I am your God.
I will strengthen you and help you;
　　I will uphold you with my righteous right
　　hand.

Isaiah 41:10

The ride home from the doctor's office that day was eerily quiet; both of us were lost in our own thoughts and too emotionally drained to form anything remotely resembling a sentence. We returned to the house on Dauphin Avenue that we had just left hours earlier. Now even our once cozy safe haven offered no shelter from the onslaught of unknowns. We limped through the week, feeling as though we had just been dropped off in a foreign land of uncharted territory where we didn't even speak the language. We were utterly lost, praying each day for guidance and direction. Thankfully, within days, we slowly began to feel God's grace warming our cold stone fear. It was if we were now pioneers in that uncharted land, standing in the cool waters, sifting millions of grains of sandy sediment in search of that one tiny shimmering nugget of gold, the promise of a bright tomorrow.

During that process of soul searching and acceptance, Jon and I sat at Thanksgiving dinner at my parents' house trying to answer our family's concerned inquiries without causing too much alarm. We simply announced that we were once again expecting at least twins. Everyone was elated that we had indeed managed to get pregnant, clearly not knowing in the least the myriad of emotions that bubbled just below the surface.

As dessert was passed and the excited talk of babies turned to the ebb and flow of familiar small talk, Jon and I reached the first of many milestones in our newfound destiny. Although we knew we saw the circles on the screen, all seven of them, we still clung to the hope that just maybe some of them wouldn't be there next time. Regardless, whatever God chose to give us, we would accept as a blessing. It was Thanksgiving, and we were thankful.

My newfound thankfulness was quickly put to the test the very next day, Black Friday, as it is referred to in the retail world. As millions of people scurried from store to store hoping for bargains that would make someone on their freshly written Christmas list very happy, I was once again having cold gel smeared all over my already enlarging belly in preparation for yet another ultrasound. Grasping at any reassuring thought he could think of, Jon, half laughing, or maybe half choking, quipped as we made our way to our appointment, "It's pretty bad when you're praying for quads."

God answered those prayers — and then some!

We studied the screen intently and soon zeroed in on the four embryonic sacks that had previously been noted as "occupied." They did indeed contain tiny beating hearts snuggled deep within each bubble-shaped abode. However, an additional two pulsating specks drummed as steadily as a dripping faucet in the still of night. There they were — all of our worst fears at the wildest odds — blinking on the screen, hammering in the reality with each breathtaking stroke. Six babies. Just six. It was not only that we were too overwhelmed, too exhausted, and too numb to panic, but actually that our resolve to deal with this revelation as thankfully as possible had already kicked in and our testimony had begun.

That's not to say we instantly fell into a state of parental bliss. Each and every day brought a new set of questions and challenges — psychological, physical, and financial dilemmas. I quickly faced almost unbearable changes in my body. I was extremely nauseated, utterly exhausted, had already given up working, and, although it was still early in my first trimester, on complete bed rest.

A "normal" day at seven weeks found me lying on the couch in the family room with my toddler girls chattering and busily playing around me. We would play games like "restaurant" where I would send one twin scampering off to the refrigerator to fill my yogurt order while the other one retrieved the spoon. I would sleepily watch as they lined up their soft baby dolls, pretending to feed and clothe them, lovingly mothering them. I tried to imagine as I looked at the vast array of plastic toes and fingers how I would possibly feed, change, and care for that many real babies at once.

I once overheard Mady, at the ripe old age of three, dramatically telling Cara in her most exhausted pretend voice that she "had to go lie down because of the sextuplets." I realized that my girls in their happy pretend world had already begun to deal with our topsy-turvy real world—and by God's grace, they were doing just fine. They were young enough to not really know any differently, yet mature enough to vocalize what they were feeling.

I was blessed to have help three mornings a week from a kind woman named Ruth, whom Jon's dad had graciously volunteered to hire. The girls looked forward to a new audience to entertain, and I eagerly anticipated the few hours of quiet followed by naptime for both the girls and me.

I also allowed them for the very first time since they were born to ride in a car other than one driven by Jon or me. A friend and neighbor offered to take them for an outing to the library once a week. This decision for me was huge. Remember, I was a bit of a control freak, and to allow my precious girls to be out of my sight involved a loosening of the apron strings that I was not at all accustomed to doing. As I watched them dance in the front door after their first adventure to the exciting book-lined shelves of our local library, I realized that God was surely succeeding in teaching me the first of many difficult lessons. I might have always thought I was in control, that those girls were mine, but He was saying, "No, Kate, they are mine first. I love them even more than you ever possibly could. Let me be in control!" It was with a lump in my throat and surrender in my heart that I finally relinquished control of not only my toddlers, but also my six unborn children to the almighty God who made the vast universe and who could most certainly watch over my suddenly expanding family.

●

With all that time on the couch, my head reeled with the many tasks that needed to be done for Christmas, which was quickly approaching. My handy pint-sized assistants brought me pen and paper on which I determinedly scribbled a detailed Christmas list of all the items that had been on my original "to-do" list but had been forgotten weeks ago. I then proceeded to call in the troops in the form of family and friends who came to my rescue and shopped till they dropped. Once again God was whispering a lesson. He was teaching me that although I had always been so proud of standing on my own two feet and being extremely self-sufficient and self-reliant, I was now going to need to swallow my pride and ask for help. It was for the sake of my family. They needed me to be sane, healthy, and strong—not just in control.

The dark days of winter crept on. Besides looking forward to the holidays, I was also warily awaiting my next doctor's appointment at 8:00 a.m. on Christmas Eve. I was scheduled to have a peripherally inserted central catheter, or PICC line, inserted into my left arm. This intravenous line would allow me to administer fluids to myself at home and hopefully eliminate, or at least reduce, my too frequent hospital visits due to dehydration. Although the actual insertion process is, let's just say, less than enjoyable, I was eager to have the procedure done. I had specifically requested it in my quest to be as independent as possible for as long as possible.

By that time I was seeing a new doctor in Hershey, Pennsylvania. Due to the fact that I required the most modern facilities and expertise that a large hospital offers, I had had the choice of either Philadelphia or Hershey. I chose the latter due to the fact that Hershey is less than an hour's drive from home with far less traffic. The biggest factor, however, was Dr. Botti. After our initial conversation with that humble man, I knew that he was the one to help me along this winding pothole-riddled road to delivery. He is kind and brilliant, but more important, he seemed to understand that he was just an instrument being used by the Great Physician to see that both my babies and I were given the best possible chance at survival.

Before the appointment, we had decided to stay overnight with my parents who live in the peaceful Pennsylvania countryside not far from the Penn State Milton S. Hershey Medical Center. It would be a nice reprieve from our daily routine, and the girls loved any sort of outing, soaking in the attention and relishing what they perceived to be a mini adventure.

Suddenly, our festive pre-holiday visit abruptly shifted gears. I woke in the middle of the night feeling what no pregnant woman in her first trimester wants to feel—a tremendous surge of fluid that could only mean something was terribly wrong. Fighting to remain calm, I just lay quietly in bed, looking at the pale light of the moon on the ceiling and praying with all my might that I was just imagining things. Eventually I got up the nerve to slide onto a small bedside commode that my mother had thoughtfully placed nearby for me to use.

As soon as I noticed the unfathomable amount of fresh blood, I just screamed and kept screaming. Jon, of course, shot straight up from bed and leaped into action, calling my mother and the nurse care line for my doctor, which was frustratingly busy for almost a full hour. We were told to get to the emergency room immediately. My worried mother shoved a stack of 3 x 5 white index cards into my quivering hand as we hastily opened her front door and stepped out into the frigid country air.

Upon arrival at the hospital, we created quite a stir as we desperately stumbled over our hurried words trying to explain that I was carrying sextuplets. It took more than one attempt, as several confused nurses thought I was saying that I already had six children. Once they finally realized my frail and unusual condition, I was taken to a comparatively quiet room, still in the emergency department, where all I remember saying over and over again was, "Please do an ultrasound. Please!"

The brusque doctor who had been called in to examine me quickly summed up the chaotic situation and sharply called for a plastic collection cup. As a nurse I knew that meant that she felt I was having a miscarriage and needed to collect tissue to verify its content.

A wave of emotion struck me like an icy winter blast. After weeks of coming to terms with my risky pregnancy, of dealing with the roller coaster ride of ups and downs, of finally grasping some form of acceptance, I felt it all slipping away. I sobbed with sorrow and grief that this crazy, painful drama would all be coming to an end just as Jon and I were feeling ready to deal with it. I felt a strength rise up in me like the fury of a mother bear. I wanted these babies, and I was ready to fight for them.

I demanded that the doctor allow me to see the contents of the cup, and after much verbal volleying, she reluctantly surrendered it for my inspection. With not only a nurse's training but also a mother's instinct, I was clearly convinced that there was no tissue in the cup, and I demanded to see Dr. Botti. Finally, after what seemed like hours, I was put on the phone with my obstetrician, and I begged once more for an ultrasound to be performed. He calmly reassured me that he would send his own technicians directly to the hospital, and they would perform the ultrasound as soon as possible. Thank goodness! I finally felt like someone was listening.

After what seemed like an eternity, I once again lay on a cold table in a dimly lit room. I painstakingly positioned myself to get a clear view of the ultrasound screen that would report the happenings of my uterus like an exclusive riveting report on the evening news. My thoughts were so intent that I first heard the focused technician as if from a distance. "I see six."

"What?" I gasped. "Jon, did she say six?" I begged for confirmation. More than anything in the world, just like any other pregnant mother, I wanted my babies to be okay, to be safe and secure in their dark snug den in the depths of my being.

I heard my husband reply. "I counted too, Kate. Six hearts."

I gratefully sobbed, "Thank You, Lord; thank You, Lord; they're all still there!" From that moment on, everyone around us felt the electricity, the emotion, and I believe the almighty hand of God. A 180-degree change in expectations and attitudes occurred, and everyone was now pulling for the babies as a team. We were no longer feeling the negative draw of statistics but the positive truth that "with God all things are possible." To this day, Jon and I refer to that night as our "Christmas Miracle."

Early the following morning, I kept my scheduled appointment and proceeded to have the PICC line inserted. It was a long day, to say the least. How does one recover from such a horrendous twenty-four hours? Jon and I were quick to learn it is by just putting one foot in front of the other, praying hard with each step. And that is what we did.

We returned home to Wyomissing late on Christmas Eve. Once inside, Jon tended to the task of helping me into bed for the night while the girls chirped about the events of the day, asking rapid-fire questions peppered with sporadic reminders of what the next morning would bring. As I lay in bed reviewing the dramatic events of the day, I felt very alone and isolated as I listened to what sounded like a squirmy, squealing wrestling match on the floor above me — involving two freshly bathed charmers with matching footed pajamas and one very patient daddy.

I felt sorry for myself as that monster "Why me?" question trudged around and around in my head. I regretted that I had completely missed a Christmas Eve in my young daughters' lives after having spent weeks anticipating Mady's and Cara's smiles on their first year of really understanding the true meaning of Christmas. I felt like I had somehow cheated them of having both parents tuck them into their warm beds after having had teeth brushed, a book read, and the whole "visions of sugarplums" idea refreshed in their minds.

Changes were coming fast and furious. On that melancholy night, I realized that my personal involvement in every memory-making moment of their lives was among the first of many selfless sacrifices Mady and Cara would learn to make in order to hold the high honor of becoming big sisters to six younger siblings. I, lover of predictability and despiser of change, was also reminded yet again that our old way of tradition and order would be shattered to pieces. Like reflections in a broken mirror, our new life would need to be carefully replaced piece by piece before we began to recognize any resemblance to our old description of "family."

The holiday came and went with Jon taking charge of all of the related festivities and his mother filling in the gaps. Meanwhile, I languished on the couch trying to stay upbeat and positive as January made its wintry debut.

At approximately fourteen weeks, I had the stretched round belly of what would normally be considered that of a woman who was maybe seven months along. I hurt. Everything hurt as my body struggled to comprehend and make allowance for the immense job it was being called to do. Most days involved a tremendous amount of faith and mental tenacity with a touch of sheer stubbornness just to maintain my sanity. I spent hours shuffling through the already dog-eared 3 x 5 cards that my mother had given me weeks earlier during my traumatic stay at her house. On each card she had handwritten a Scripture that would encourage me and remind me that the God I served was an almighty, loving, kind, and generous God who would provide every breath I needed, just as He always had.

My aches and pains were so widespread and so often that when I felt a "strange" pain one January night during my tenth trip to the bathroom, I simply wrote it off as probably another unexplainable side effect of my unusual pregnancy. I didn't yet realize that the ringmaster's bell had rung and I was in for another round of thrashing blows to my already battered body. The unwavering barrage of all-consuming pain persisted as once again the hospital personnel scrambled to find its source and carefully considered all the extraordinary medical facts of my situation. The assisting nurse mercifully administered an injection of pain killing Demerol while the doctor eventually concluded that I had passed a kidney stone. I breathed a deep sigh of relief as my space-crunching crew of babies and I had evaded yet another scare, and I would be free to go home and resume my post on the couch.

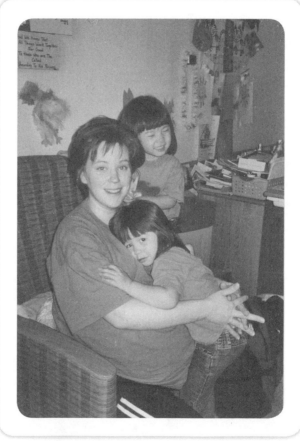

*Comforting Cara during a visit with Mommy
in the hospital. Notice the verses and
cards that lined the walls.*

5 The Hard Work of Rest

"Come to me, all you who are weary and burdened,
and I will give you rest."

Matthew 11:28

Once upon a time, when I heard the term *bed rest*, I conjured up a picture of a blissful mom-to-be propped up in her cozy king-sized bed on freshly laundered sheets, surrounded by ten down pillows situated just right. The sweet song of bluebirds nesting in the branches of the nearest blossoming cherry tree would be heard drifting in through her open bedroom window on a bright and sunny spring day. Her cheerful husband would sweep into the room with a tray beautifully set with a nicely grilled filet mignon, steaming baked potato, fresh organic veggies, and a large frosty chocolate shake. Also on the tray would be a sweet-smelling rose and her favorite magazines to peruse at her leisure. She would be smiling, showered, and serene, with her hand resting lightly on the healthy bump under her stylish maternity dress, a gift from one of her many and frequent caring visitors.

I don't have that picture anymore. That bubble burst and left one tired, scared, uncomfortable pincushion in the middle of reality.

My days of bed rest began by checking and documenting my weight and blood pressure. I was then required to wear a fetal monitor for at least one hour each morning and then again one hour in the evening. The machine would send via the phone lines all of the day's events in my busy uterus to the nurse on duty. She would eventually call back to either give the okay or say, "Get to the hospital."

I also gave myself injections of Heparin twice a day, which was prescribed to ward off any blood clots. I would ice the chosen spot for that day, but still I was quickly covered with angry black and blue marks.

I had no time to dwell on bruises, however; I had to care for the subcutaneous terbutaline pump in my upper thigh. That's really just a fancy name for a small device that looks like a thumbtack stuck in your body, which you are supposed to pretend doesn't bother you at all. The medicine being administered through it was to decrease and hopefully even prevent contractions. I was to check the site daily, and after three days remove it, restring the new tubing, and reinsert it in a different spot. I still cringe just thinking about it, not only because it was obviously a despised nuisance but unfortunately didn't work. The medicine left me feeling jittery and dizzy as my heart rate raced to 150 beats per minute. I was able to keep the pump set at a low grade, but so low that it never reached a level that was deemed helpful.

At eighteen weeks, I could barely bend over, and the strain of caring for the girls and me was taking its toll on Jon. To add to our mounting pile of stress, Jon was called into the office of the plant where he worked, accused of "stealing time" from the company, and given his pink slip.

Six weeks previously, Jon had told his employers of the situation with the babies because, when the grace period for my insurance expired after I stopped working, the babies would be added to the health insurance plan provided through his company. The company was immediately concerned that their premiums would "go through the roof." Although it was later intimated in a court hearing that the impending expenses of insurance for premature sextuplets was indeed a factor in Jon being fired, Jon still lost the hearing.

In just two months' time, we went from a very comfortable two-salary family to a couple who was quickly running out of strength, energy, and now savings. It was a major blow to our dwindling living expenses as well as to our fragile egos. We had both worked extremely hard and managed our money wisely, and yet we feared we would be looked upon as slackers in our bustling community of American dream seekers. We didn't want sympathy. We didn't want handouts. We really just wanted our family to survive—literally. We knew we were going to need to redefine what our basic needs were and stretch every last penny, learning to budget in areas that we thought were already tightly budgeted.

During that same time, my doctor decided it was finally time that I was admitted to the hospital where I would remain under close observation until the birth of the babies. I chose the much-feared date: March 7. I would be just twenty weeks pregnant. That gave us exactly two weeks to prepare both ourselves and the girls for a heart-wrenching departure and a lengthy separation. I was dreading it. How do you explain to three-year-olds that Mommy won't be home for a couple months; and then when she finally does get home, she will have a smaller tummy but a much bigger heart swollen with love for eight children, not just two? The girls curiously listened as I read my hospital list to Jon's dad, their Poppy, who was always more than willing to help us with our errands. The girls then helped Jon pack my few belongings—a huge shower towel, a scrunchie with a long handle so I could wash without bending over, pretty purple and blue sheets, and of course some of their very own artwork.

A few nights before I left, we decided that we would splurge on something I had been wildly craving for weeks—crab legs and ribs from a local restaurant called The Crab Barn. We referred to it as our Last Supper, although to be fair, it was more accurately my Last Supper. Jon tried to swipe a stray crab leg or two, but—what can I say? I was really hungry! Nevertheless, we both look back on that night with warm memories of the last private moments we would have as a couple for a very long time.

It wasn't until years later that we realized God had always had a plan when Jon lost his job. He knew that Jon was needed at home during those difficult weeks. Because he was home, we were able to prepare; I was able to leave for the hospital knowing that Mady and Cara would have their daddy taking good care of them. It's unimaginable to think what we would have done had Jon not been able to stay with the girls. It was a season of our lives that seemed like a nightmare while we were experiencing it; however, with the wisdom of hindsight, we realized it was yet another blessing, a lesson in trusting that God sees to the details. I can't even count the number of times since then that I have lived that truth.

March 7 quietly dawned gray and damp, a Sunday that looked like any other late winter day — except for us, it was the much talked

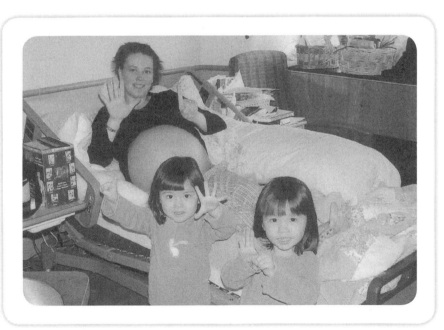

Hospital bed rest.

about "Mommy's going to the hospital" day. Jon thoughtfully laid out warm blankets in the back of our white minivan, because by then I could not sit up for the hour-long drive to the Penn State Milton S. Hershey Medical Center where our babies would eventually be born. I listened to Mady and Cara chatter in their car seats, the tops of their heads just barely visible to me from my makeshift bed. With a brave face we said our good-byes to a few friends from church who had visited to share a pizza and pray with us before we left for the hospital. As I watched out the back window at our little house staring blankly back at me, I wondered how it was possible that I could feel so enormous and bulky and yet at the same time so very small and helpless. I tried desperately to imprint the memory of our neighborhood on my mind. I knew it would be many months before I returned.

I arrived at my new "home away from home," anxious and already claustrophobic. To my great relief, my mom, knowing that I am a manic germophobe, arrived at my room on the labor and delivery floor armed with Clorox wipes and antibacterial soap. She immediately got down to business and meticulously cleaned every surface until it emanated the refreshing scent of a summer breeze rather than the usual medicinal smelling industrial spray. Jon and the nurses scurried around the room making the bed, fluffing pillows, and hanging my three-year-olds' colorful masterpieces on the bulletin board that faced the bed. The nurses were so proud to tell me how they had even managed to finagle me a room with a view. Outside my one window lay a beautiful peaceful field where the deer were known to frequently visit in hopes of finding a mid-winter snack. Later, I would stare out that window for weeks and weeks, loving the languid, graceful beauty of my daily visitors.

This day, however, I sat feeling wretchedly round, somewhat useless, and disturbingly breathless. Scanning the room I suddenly had a flashback to my freshman year of college. I recalled how I had felt having to adjust to a whole new way of life, a whole new routine where I had limited living space and overwhelming responsibility. I didn't know anyone and felt strange and uneasy—displaced.

In the small quarters of my hospital room, I even wondered if this is what it felt like to be in prison. I know I sound like I'm being a bit melodramatic, but I understood very clearly that I was not going to be lying around in the lap of luxury. Plus, my bulging girth was every bit as effective as the sturdiest shackles. I begged pathetically for the nurse to "find the man" who might be able to figure out a way to open my hospital room window. I so desperately needed to breathe the fresh air and feel a brisk breeze.

Although everyone was doing their best to make my stay more bearable, I had an inescapable lead role on this new team of miracle-seekers. I was expected to adhere to a strict set of guidelines that were to be taken extremely seriously if I was going to carry the babies for at least another ten weeks. One of those guidelines was to consume at least four thousand calories every day. The plan consisted of three meals, three snacks, and three six-hundred-calorie shakes. At one time in my life, that order would've made me think I had died and gone to heaven. Unfortunately, as good as it sounds and as hard as I tried, none of the food I was consuming would stay down for very long. I had such miserable acid reflux, that shortly after a meal, I would vomit violently. It was as if my squished and rebelling stomach were burning hot with anger and vehemently protesting one more ounce of space-hogging food.

One of the most horrid experiences of my hospital stay was when I awoke in the middle of the night spewing what felt like gallons of searing acid from both my mouth and nose. Wide-eyed, groping, and gasping for help, I felt as if I were drowning. I was quickly put on an IV of Reglan and Zantac, and from then on could not eat anything after eight o'clock at night. The episode burned my vocal cords, leaving me with a rasping sore throat for two weeks.

To aid in my ever so difficult quest for food, Dr. Botti allowed me to order my daily meals from the employee menu. It certainly wasn't a four-star restaurant, but at least it was a bit tastier than the normal hospital fare. I remember one day he strolled happily into my room for his morning visit holding a nice fat candy bar. Handing it to me he said, "Nobody else can eat a candy bar before eleven o'clock in the morning, but you can." I happened to be in Hershey, Pennsylvania, home of the famous Hershey bar, so I'm pretty sure I was not the first person to sample some of the area's finest at the crack of dawn. And anyway, who was I to argue with my brilliant and always caring doctor?

Speaking of arguing, I did have one major dispute in the first week of my hospital stay. Jon and I would later dub the disturbing three-day standoff between me and the hospital administration "The Vitamin Wars." Having read up on all the essential vitamins and nutrients a pregnant woman's body demands, since day one of my pregnancy I had been taking several supplements, namely a good quality multivitamin, vitamin C, calcium, magnesium, cod liver oil, and a very large dose of folic acid. When I was admitted, I was told that I could not take anything from home that was not prescribed by my doctor. Being in somewhat precarious and uncharted waters, I knew they were concerned that adding yet another variable to my already complicated case could potentially muddy the waters. On the other hand, I was convinced that I had made it as far as I had at least in part due to my dedication in giving my body those extra vitamins it so desperately craved. I felt so strongly about my stance that I eventually threatened to check myself out of the hospital if I were not given permission to continue with my well-engrained routine. Thankfully, the hospital finally relented and agreed to the vitamins.

That small victory was a momentary bright spot in an otherwise bleak and lonely week. Just one day after I was admitted, Jon and both of the girls suffered a terrible bout of the flu. They could not visit me until they completely recovered due to the high risk of passing on what could potentially be a devastating illness to someone in my condition. It lasted a very long seven days, and I missed them beyond description.

My next dilemma was my skin. I was quickly beginning to show early signs of bedsores, a painful condition that often plagues bed-ridden patients. At twenty-one weeks, my belly measured forty-two centimeters in circumference. Needless to say, I was not overly mobile. Once again my knight in shining scrubs, Dr. Botti, came to my rescue. He prescribed an ICU bed that would allow me to change my position more easily and more often. Along with that order came the stern ban on all night nurses in my room between the hours of ten o'clock at night and seven o'clock in the morning. Alleluia! With all of the kicking and shoving of six little night owls, I really didn't need any more distractions when and if I finally did get comfortable enough to sleep.

My days eventually settled into a routine. I thought in a meal-to-meal, snack-to-snack kind of way. Ironically, much like a determined dieter is practically obsessed with the prospect of her next meal, I thought of, but dreaded, every meal. I had zero stomach capacity and my appetite was virtually nonexistent. As difficult as it was, however, I was fiercely devoted to the daunting task of supplying my children with as many calories as I could possibly keep down.

My mother would visit me for at least one hour every day, which was always a welcome break. She would fill my ice bucket, bring me occasional treats, and generally try to encourage me. She also had the all-important task of hanging that day's entire array of cards. She knew I eagerly anticipated the arrival of the mailman as he breezed into my room every afternoon with my stack of mail. Initially I would tear through them in just minutes. Later I realized that like a fine wine, mail time was meant to be savored. As I got more and more disciplined, spacing my letter-opening over several hours, they would provide small reassuring hugs throughout an entire day. This was just another way of learning to cope with a whole lot of hours and nowhere to go.

I was also extremely grateful for Jon's father who supplied calling cards from Sam's Club with enough minutes to keep in touch with the daily happenings at home as well as to laugh, cry, pray, or just chat with some supportive friends from both near and far away. He also supplied a laptop computer with a webcam. What a technological miracle to be able to see and talk to my two growing pixies from forty-five miles away. Amazing!

Another momentous gift was given to me in the form of a massage. A considerate, generous friend, Susan, who had given me a prenatal massage once a week at home beginning at fifteen weeks, volunteered to drive to Hershey twice a week — and three times a week right before delivery — to continue with her gentle healing ministry. She shared with me the belief that massage therapy during pregnancy is known to improve circulation, reduce discomfort, relieve mental fatigue, and generally enhance the physiological and emotional well-being of both the mother and her baby. How can I ever thank someone enough who gave of herself so freely and willingly to give my babies a better chance of survival? She also gave me something to look forward to each week. I couldn't wait to see her peek her head in my door. Susan, knowing how much I valued that restorative hour, would put a sign on my door saying, "Massage in progress." To this day, I believe that the gift of her massage played an important role in my body's ability to hold on, one day at a time.

On Monday, March 15, I listened with tears in my eyes as I heard the pitter-patter of four little feet scampering down the hall. The girls had fully recovered from the flu, and I would finally see them. As they walked through the door, I remember thinking how much older Cara had gotten in just a little over a week. She looked so much taller.

The girls were always a bit unsure as to what they were supposed to do in that sterile room while Mommy tried desperately to soak up the sight and smell of them for just a while longer. They generally told me funny stories, taking turns to fill in the details as twins often do. Cara once commented with innocent sincerity that "a house is not the same without a mommy in it." Tears immediately formed in my eyes. Then there were other moments that brought a smile to my face. One such time was when Mady pressed her outstretched hand on the upper-left side of my belly, and for the first time, felt Baby D give her a good kick. Mady jumped back and said, "Oooooh," with a look of surprise and wonder.

Sometimes the occupational therapist would leave toys in my room knowing my girls would welcome the stimulation and distraction. She also would bring me art supplies so I could prepare a craft project that we could tackle together when they arrived. I was never quite certain if those projects were for the girls' entertainment or if she gave me all that cutting and gluing as a simple boredom buster. Either way, it worked quite nicely.

At twenty-two weeks, indocin was prescribed to relax my uterus. It was not unusual for me to begin contracting mildly almost every night. Unfortunately, the medicine added to my acid reflux problem and, even worse, carried a risk of reducing the babies' amniotic fluid. To monitor that fluid, I was given daily ultrasounds. As uncomfortable and bothersome as the constant pressing and prodding became, I generally looked forward to those few minutes of reassurance, seeing that my babies were all present and accounted for. Listening to the steady drum of each little heart gave me just enough of an energy boost to plod through some otherwise bleak days.

The growth of each baby was also carefully calculated and documented every two weeks. I was constantly amazed as I observed the latest technology reveal the length of a delicate femur, the circumference of a skull, the chambers of a heart. I watched and listened carefully during these intense measuring visits with my babies.

I would quietly cheer each one on as he or she stepped up to the scrutiny of the technician's wand. It gave me tremendous motherly pride to see that my babies grew with great team spirit. There were no slackers, no one lagging behind. Each baby was usually within several ounces of the others, and even while living in some pretty tight quarters, each appeared to be thriving and growing. I would heartily congratulate each one for logging a few more precious ounces in our weight journal.

I also firmly reminded each one that our goal was thirty-two weeks. Back at twenty-four weeks, we rejoiced in a viability celebration of a game well played, but there was still so much work to be done; endurance and sheer will were necessary to net a few more goals before we could claim a victory. "Thirty-two weeks, thirty-two weeks!" became my insistent chant.

Another marvelous perk of the frequent ultrasounds was, of course, the inside scoop on the sex of the babies. It was hard to imagine that just one generation ago, mothers had not the faintest idea what secrets their body held; yet, there I was with a front-row seat and X-ray vision.

I had learned at just eighteen weeks that our "team" had even sides; we were expecting three girls and three boys. Jon and I were ecstatic! Three girls and three boys had a nice symmetrical feel to it. Jon's first comment was, "Great! They can take each other to the prom." He was, in his own abstract way of thinking, just trying to protect his girls, though I thought maybe he was jumping ahead just a bit too fast. I concentrated, of course, on the more practical things: We could more easily divide them for bedrooms someday — now I was the one jumping ahead as I thought of our cramped little house where all six babies would share one bedroom. Plus, the even split avoided some of the issues that might arise from, say, five girls and one boy. Can you imagine? A grand total of seven girls pit against one token male to carry the Gosselin name.

Jon and I had chosen names fairly early in my pregnancy, as both of us found it surprisingly easy to agree. Maybe it wasn't that surprising since we did have six opportunities to add our personal favorites. We decided, not yet knowing the sexes, that we would choose—yes, you guessed it—three girls' names and three boys' names. Our only rule was that names put down for discussion had to be definitely boy or definitely girl. Our life was going to be confusing enough without having a future helper not know if I was asking her to bring me a boy or a girl. Our reason for deciding on three names each was that we were assured of having at least a few of them work depending on the sexes of the babies. I still giggle that our God, knowing I needed to have at least something checked off the list, would allow us to think of the exact number of necessary names. It was just another confirmation to me that He knew each and every one of them by name before I even knew who they were. I am still amazed!

Alexis and Aaden were our first choices. We had chosen those two names way before even planning a second pregnancy. We agreed that we would go alphabetically, and therefore the two *A* names would be for the first girl and boy to be delivered. It was more difficult to agree on the spelling of Aaden however. Jon rallied feverishly for A-i-d-e-n. I wanted A-a-d-e-n. I guess you can figure out who won that one!

The next baby to be named was Collin. We chose the name because Mady had asked for a baby brother named Collin before I was even pregnant. Where a three-year-old even heard of that name is still a mystery! But in typical Mady fashion, she was pretty persistent, so we agreed.

Hannah was a simple decision. I had been lying on the couch in the family room, which was several steps below the hallway that led from the living room to the kitchen. As I spotted Jon walk by, I yelled up, "Hey, what about Hannah?" He was probably busy making dinner or rounding up the girls for their bath, but he hesitated just for an instant and yelled back, "Yep, I like it!"

"H on the end?" I shouted back.

"Yep!" came the quick Jon-like response.

Somewhere in the naming process I remembered something from a visit at my grandparents' church. A couple in the church had adopted a petite Asian baby girl whom they had named Leah. I smiled as I recalled her sweet and fragile "China doll" appearance. Envisioning a tiny Leah of my own, I happily wrote the third girl's name on our final list after Jon agreed.

We needed one more boy's name. I had always wanted a Joey — not Joseph, just Joey. Jon couldn't picture this little Asian kid running around with an Italian-sounding name. I guess he did have a point. Eventually I had a brainstorm: I came up with the name Joel, thinking of someone I had once known whose name was Joel but whom everyone referred to as Joey. It was perfect! (Joey never did take hold, but as our Joel later toddled around with his silly snickering grin, Joely seemed to fit just right!)

With all six names fittingly chosen, we turned our attention to the middle names. I had made a promise to God that if I was ever blessed with another daughter, that Faith would be used in her name to always remind me of the all important role our faith had played in bringing her to fruition. So, the first baby girl to be born, Alexis, came to be Alexis Faith. I loved it and thought it sounded so pretty. It made me think of a favorite Bible passage, Galatians 5:22–23: "But the fruit of the Spirit is love, joy, peace, longsuffering, kindness, goodness, faithfulness, gentleness, self-control" (NKJV). Those were definitely the characteristics I desperately prayed my daughters would someday possess. We decided to use that peaceful theme to weave our girls together in a common bond of godly goals.

Mulling over the depth of that verse, I felt "Joy" jump out at me as the next choice for a middle name. I tried it with Hannah, saying aloud, 'Hannah Joy, Hannah Joy." It seemed so natural. Perfect.

Next came Leah. Wanting to stay with the theme, I was a little worried when I realized that while longsuffering and self-control were definitely admirable traits, neither were suitable middle names! Fortunately, as I lay on bed rest, one word kept coming to mind: hope. Hope was the number one thing that filled my days. That was it! Leah Hope. It gave me chills and I knew we had a winner. I was thrilled that I would always be able to tell my girls that faith and hope got us here, and they will bring us a lot of joy!

For the boys' middle names, we went the more traditional route and looked to our family tree for inspiration. Aaden was named Aaden Jonathan after his daddy, and Collin became Collin Thomas after Jon's father. Once again we were faced with a tougher decision when it came to naming Joel. (Sorry, Joel!) I had originally liked Joel Michael after a baby I used to babysit when I was young. However, that wasn't in keeping with the family line of thinking that we had used for the other two boys. I didn't want our Joel to feel excluded, and I also very much wanted to honor my brother Kevin. I ran the name Joel Kevin past Jon. He said, "Last boy ever, last chance ever. It works. Yes." He had consolidated my long rambling reasonings down to ten words or less — one of his skills I find equally handy and annoying, depending on the situation. In this case, it sealed the deal and Joel Kevin it was.

The most satisfying part of naming Joel though was keeping the secret from my brother. He had called to check in with me one day, and I casually told him that I had changed one of the baby's names. He really wasn't interested in what most men would consider trivial information when compared to football scores and what was for dinner. So when I chattered on about wanting a family name rather than Michael for Joel, I could almost see Kevin's eyes glaze over through the telephone line. Finally, I ended with, "and so we would like his name to be Joel Kevin, after you!"

I heard a loud moment of silence, a mumbled something, and then we ended our call and hung up. I sat thinking about how odd that was when not two minutes later, the phone on the nightstand rang again. It was Kevin. "Kate, that's really cool. Thanks. I'm honored!" I realized it had taken Kevin a few minutes to process the fact that he would now have a miniature namesake who would have a forever bond with his Uncle Kevin.

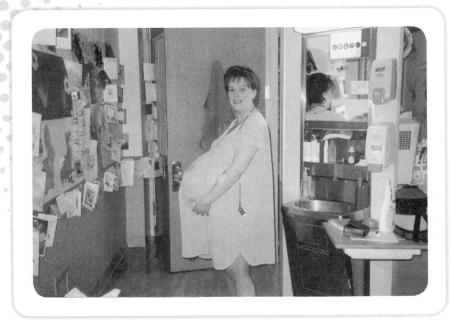

Delivery day: May 10, 2004. Kate at 54 inches around.

6 Media Mayhem

To everything there is a season,
    A time for every purpose under heaven ...
    A time to keep silence,
And a time to speak.

Ecclesiastes 3:1, 7 NKJV

It was everyone's fear that once I had been admitted to the hospital the news of our unusual adventure would leak to the media. Dr. Botti warned us that the birth of sextuplets would most definitely lead to a media feeding frenzy and that there was probably no way to avoid at least some of it. However, he also wisely advised both of us to keep our story as quiet as possible until I was at least twenty-four weeks along, the first magic number for those women eking out each day of a difficult pregnancy. It is the point where most doctors consider a baby to be viable with at least a 50/50 chance of survival.

I loved that Dr. Botti — thorough, wise, and discerning — was willing to shield us under the umbrella of the hospital's care, wanting to alleviate as much stress as possible from our already too-full plate. Besides taking my name off my door and making it clear to hospital staff that he would not tolerate undue stress put upon his patient, he even went so far as to make Jon look him in the eye and promise that he would do everything in his power to shield me from the press for the sake of our babies' well-being. Jon wholeheartedly agreed, and it was decided that when the time came to speak to the media, Jon would act as spokesperson for both of us, for all of us.

He would not have to go it alone, however. The hospital assigned a public relations liaison named Amy Buehler-Stranges. She was a tall, thin, soft-spoken young woman who handled her pressure-packed job with strength and clarity. She was the person we trusted to eventually smooth the path when it was confirmed that Jon would be present at a news conference announcing our precious news to the general public.

On Monday, April 5, Jon took his seat in the middle of a long banquet table. He was accompanied by Dr. Botti, Dr. Mujsce, head of neonatology, along with the head nurse of my unit, and Dr. Repke, the head of obstetrics and gynecology. Cameras flashed and the panel of seasoned professionals and one very proud daddy-to-be fielded scores of questions from a room packed full of eager reporters. It was officially announced that Jon and I were indeed expecting six babies and we hoped they would make their appearance between thirty and thirty-two weeks. Jon happily revealed the sexes of our babies, three girls and three boys, followed by the names that we had chosen for each of them. Amy was present of course, overseeing all of the many details, and the pastor of our church at that time came to offer moral support for Jon.

It was excruciating to sit confined in my room while my husband faced his first test of public attention. I felt like it was a rite of passage in a sense that we were now telling the world that the birth of sextuplets might actually happen. Even if they had been born the next day, God forbid, the reality was that they at least had some chance of survival. I was beaming with pride at how calm, cool, and collected Jon appeared to be in spite of it all. My mom later called to say that the girls had watched Daddy on television. We laughed together as she explained how the girls had shrieked in unison when they realized whom they were watching.

In addition to that first press conference, Jon and I had agreed to give our hometown newspaper, the *Reading Eagle*, an in-room exclusive interview. It was really sort of a self-defense move as a result of information that we had received several weeks earlier. Supposedly someone who had worked with me at the Reading Hospital was threatening to go to the press. In an attempt to buy us those few precious weeks that Dr. Botti desired, we agreed to the exclusive interview when the timing was right. But other than that one interview, thankfully no other reporters were allowed in my room.

Making our announcement official served to officially open the floodgates. Suddenly Jon and I noticed strange things happening, like random people standing at my door trying to get a peek inside. Physicians I had never met before starting stopping in to see me. We began to get calls for interviews and details.

With me getting more and more physically uncomfortable, I had no patience for the extra annoyance. My mind was preoccupied with food as eating became nearly impossible due to such weight and pressure on my stomach. I felt guilty if I couldn't eat, knowing I was responsible to deliver as much nourishment as possible to my half dozen growing babies. I begged for the doctor to give me intravenous nutrition that would supply the calories I needed.

Dr. Botti thought about it and researched it for almost an entire week before finally giving his response — no. He felt it could open up one more possibility for infection to rear its nasty head and end our efforts way too early. So I continued to obsess over what I could and could not eat and left the hospital staff to fend off curious and questioning observers and reporters.

Jon, too, had bigger fish to fry than worrying about the media. Around Easter of that year, he started a new job as an information technician at a company in Reading, Pennsylvania, just minutes from where we lived. He managed to get Ruth, whom we knew from church, to come and sit with the girls on Mondays, Tuesdays, and Wednesdays. On Wednesday nights, he would pack them up and make the hour-long drive to visit me and then drop the girls off at my parents' house. I always looked forward to Wednesday nights after not having seen Mady and Cara since the previous Sunday. On Thursdays and Fridays Jon would drive back and forth to work from Hershey and then spend the weekend with the girls at my parents' house. Obviously it was hectic!

Media attention, at first, was flattering. Who wouldn't want to know that so many people were rooting for your babies to survive? But in many ways it was an added distraction that was way beyond what we were prepared to cope with. I have to say I was very happy to peek from behind my impressive belly and know that Jon, Amy, Dr. Botti, and the hospital in general were doing their best to ease us into the inevitable limelight without it blinding us completely.

7 Countdown to Six

Therefore, since we are surrounded by such a great cloud of witnesses, let us throw off everything that hinders and the sin that so easily entangles, and let us run with perseverance the race marked out for us.

Hebrews 12:1

At twenty-eight weeks I had reached my next milestone. I was well on my way to allowing hope to really take root. And I wasn't the only one. That morning Dr. Mujsce popped into my room, and for the very first time I actually detected a small glimmer in his eyes. He knew as well as I did that we were approaching the finish line. Every day that I could manage to keep my babies safely tucked in my uterus significantly decreased their risks of having life threatening problems when they were finally born. In fact, it is a general rule that for every day in utero, a premature infant will be spared two or even three days in the Neonatal Intensive Care Unit, the NICU.

One morning in the hospital I awoke to two middle-aged men in white coats and clipboards standing over me. Clearing his throat and giving his glasses a nudge, one doctor announced that he and his colleague were there to assess my mental status. I know they were concerned because I probably appeared insanely calm and almost "glazed over" in the light of all of our very real concerns.

I, too, was amazed that I was so calm. What they didn't know or understand was that the peace of God, which even I couldn't describe, had already covered over me like a security blanket. Don't get me wrong; it wasn't as if I was living in denial. I had a bazillion concerns: Would my babies live? Would I live? Would the babies be healthy? How would we all fit into our house? How many diapers a day? A week? A year? How would we ever go anywhere again as a family when our car only fit six passengers? Would Mady and Cara be overwhelmed with this crazy change in their young lives? And what about Jon? Poor Jon had more than any man should have to endure at one time. And this was just the beginning. What about clothes, food, and—oh my goodness—college? In spite of this overwhelming list that very well could have consumed me, I had already learned that when doubt and fear began to creep in, it was imperative to redirect my focus immediately. I sang, I prayed, and I read my verses. I repeatedly handed my fears and worries back to God. He in turn rewarded me with an extra dose of peace that enabled me to creep by, minute by minute. It was this exchange that defined my days and bewildered many around me.

My favorite stress reliever came in the form of three CDs given to me by a Christian bookstore close to home, Joy Book Store. The songs on those discs soothed my heart and soul as I allowed the melody to flood my room. I would expend every last ounce of oxygen I had in my joyous daily singing to my babies. I wasn't shy! I just belted out songs of reassurance and praise. I wanted my babies to hear pure and constant encouragement. Actually, now that I think of it, maybe it was unrestrained singing at the top of my lungs that brought the two nervous men in white coats to my door! Nevertheless, the words of those songs still ring in my ears, bringing tears to my eyes and a bounce to my step.

Our twenty-eight week celebration was a seventh-inning stretch; just five days later I had my first serious labor scare. I had been very uncomfortable throughout the night and, although I was sure that I was having contractions, I was also weary of the monitors and the checking, being woken up, poked, and prodded. I was just so tired. Groggy and sleepy, I decided that I would wait until morning rounds to mention the consistent tightness gripping my belly. At morning light, I realized that instead of the normal reprieve after a few hours of sleep, the contractions that were being carefully monitored were just two minutes apart.

A flurry of activity immediately followed. I was quickly whisked over to the labor and delivery floor where I could be more closely monitored. I received an injection of terbutaline (my pump had been removed a week earlier) as well as an additional 25 milligrams of indocin, double my normal dose. While I anxiously held my breath, Dr. Botti carefully checked my cervix hoping for no serious changes. He found that I was two centimeters dilated and 50 percent effaced. Normally a woman's cervix is ten centimeters dilated and 100 percent effaced, or thinned, in order to deliver.

This news warranted a phone call to Jon telling him to come to the hospital. I could read the distress in the grim faces and voices of those around me, and it only added to my fear and sadness. I was so close to our thirty-week finish line that I could almost taste it, and now it seemed all my determination would be doused. The bad news kept coming as Dr. Botti, seeking good results from the medications, checked my cervix for the second time. Unfortunately I had dilated a bit more, to two and a half centimeters. Consequently, we all, including Jon, settled in for a long night.

The only bright spot in that whole evening was having Jon spend the night by my side. Normally he would drag himself back to our girls, exhausted and spent, leaving me behind, cranky and lonely. I would sometimes longingly listen as first-time moms and their husbands cooed over their plump newborns. I became more and more jealous that they got to enjoy what seemed like such a normal bonding experience while Jon and I waded through all of our uncertainties.

The next morning, May 4, I was wheeled back to good old room number 3266 with its card crowded walls and familiar friendly view. I had successfully evaded the onset of labor and reset my stony resolve toward that thirty-week goal.

That same day, a Tuesday, I endured my last painful growth scan. I dreaded lying on my back because I couldn't breathe from the weight and struggled not to pass out. The technician had come to my room to do the ultrasound, and I cried as she apologetically pressed and pried, trying to get a peek into what was by then a sea of squiggly limbs. The results revealed some good news and some bad news. The bad news was that the baby C's fluid levels were low, though not to a critical point yet. I would be rechecked on Friday, and if the fluid was not back up to a satisfactory level, it would be decision time.

Jon and I had prayed all along that we would never be put in a position where we would have to choose to compromise the health of all of the babies for the sake of one or more struggling babies. Dr. Botti took me off all indocin, which was possibly contributing to the low fluids, in hopes of preventing that difficult dilemma. On the positive side, we were told the approximate weight of each baby. All of the babies were well over two pounds—a whopping 15 pounds 9 ounces of sons and daughters!

At Friday's ultrasound, we received the even better news that baby C's fluid levels had slightly increased. Because he was not in the danger zone and did not seem to be in distress, it still seemed safe to hold out just a little while longer. I was still having contractions and was three centimeters dilated and 75 percent effaced.

I prayed that the days would somehow go faster. It was too painful to move or even sleep due to my gargantuan size. I felt like my body was breaking down, signaling to me that I had finally pushed it too far beyond its limits. Every tissue, muscle, ligament, and bone in my body was in agreement: this just couldn't go on much longer.

Sunday, May 9, was Mother's Day. One would think I would be feeling motherly. Carrying an extra sixty-five pounds, not able to fully extend my arms around my unbelievably big belly, sick with worry, and severely sleep deprived, I was, on the contrary, one majorly miserable mama that day. Jon came to help me take a shower as my leg muscles had atrophied and I no longer could stand for even a few minutes by myself. The bigger issue, quite literally, was that I could no longer just walk into the shower. I had to carefully back myself into the stall because I wouldn't fit any other way. I felt like a giant cement truck carrying a full load and sounding a backup alarm. Not exactly the smiling picture of maternal bliss.

In spite of my ill humor, the kind nurses surprised Jon and me with lunch from Isaac's that day as a treat. I'm sure Jon was happy for the distraction because I had been busy picking fights with him all day for no reason at all. God bless him, he patiently bore the brunt of my expended patience and perseverance.

I slept fitfully that night, waking often to go to the bathroom. I was having contractions, and eventually through my sleepy haze, I realized they were a bit different. They were actually hurting more than usual. I buzzed the nurse's station for the millionth time in ten weeks, and as always, the nurse on duty came to decipher the problem and attach a monitor. We stared at the white strip that showed three regular and strong contractions in a row. Off to the phone went the nurse to call Dr. Botti.

When Dr. Botti arrived and checked me, I was three centimeters dilated and 100 percent effaced! "Well, we are going to have some babies today!" he said.

I heard myself say a very distant and matter-of-fact, "Okay." It actually took a moment for the news to sink in. But as I drew a deep breath, I, along with everyone else involved, could feel the almost palpable energy in the air. Today was the day!

●

Dr. Botti excused himself to go notify the dozens of doctors and nurses who had been on call, awaiting the go signal.

I, of course, had previously made my own plan of action for my family to be notified. I would make six phone calls beginning with the most important—Jon. It was about four o'clock in the morning when I all but shouted into the phone to my half awake husband, "Are you ready?"

I wanted to reach through the phone line and choke him when his mumbled reply was simply, "For what?"

Well, I don't know, Jon. I thought maybe we'd play a round or two of golf, paint the garage, or why not learn to skydive on such a beautiful spring morning? I didn't say any of that, of course. I calmly announced that this was the phone call we had both been waiting for. "Today is the day, Jon. Come right away!" With that, he abruptly hung up and I returned to my task of calling my mother, brother, and sisters. Those people would in turn start a phone chain notifying more distant friends and relatives.

Amy, our public relations assistant, came into my room. She reported that the entire campus was buzzing with the news that the babies would be delivered today. In fact, pink and blue balloons by the dozens were scattered everywhere outside. It brings tears to my eyes to think once again that my babies' births were being celebrated by people I never even knew. Thank you all!

As all of the necessary preparations were being made for my required cesarean section and more and more doctors and nurses trickled into the hospital, I decided that I wanted to look the best I could to greet my sweet babies. I got up shakily, put some makeup on, and took some final pictures of my belly. I knew that even I would never be able to recall exactly how amazingly big I was.

Dr. Botti came into my room once again to personally escort me to the operating room. As he wheeled me down the hall, I rejoiced, "No more Scandi shakes!" I was referring to the three vanilla flavored supplements I drank every day in an eight-ounce glass of milk. Yuck! In minutes nurses lined the hallway and started clapping as my bed passed. I felt like how a marathon runner must feel as he nears the finish line. I had run a good race, the end was in sight, and the encouraging and rowdy claps of all my caretakers were like a final shot of adrenalin.

I was extremely nervous as the nurses began to prep me for surgery. My biggest concern was that Jon had not yet arrived. Dense fog hung in the morning air, and I was worried that he would not be thinking clearly as he made the hour-long drive. Adding to my plight was the darn skinny operating table that left me holding the tremendous weight of my belly with quivering and exhausted arms. I envisioned my whole belly cracking off like an egg on the side of a frying pan if I didn't hold it upright. Finally a nurse recognized my predicament, and they somehow managed to reposition and prop me so that I was somewhat comfortable. Thank goodness!

I must have been a pathetic sight. I had my PICC line in my outstretched left arm, a regular IV in the other arm, and a jugular line in my neck. This central line was inserted as a precaution in case I would begin to hemorrhage during the surgery. In that event, they could instantly feed blood directly through my jugular vein, the largest vein in the human body. It was one of the reasons that way back at twenty-six weeks, the anesthesiologist had told me I would be put under general anesthesia for the delivery. My answer was an unequivocal, "No way! I've waited forever to hear these babies cry and I fully intend to be awake to hear them!"

So there I lay with a doctor pushing what seemed like a ridiculously large needle and thick tube into my neck. The crunching sound was reason enough to consider the procedure completely barbaric. That was the moment when I broke down and almost lost all control. Sobbing to the kind man at the head of my bed, I cried, "I've been brave and strong for so long, and I just can't do it anymore."

He tried to calm me with his soothing and gentle demeanor. "Katie, you can do this," he said.

The torture continued. Next came the spinal block. A spinal block numbs the patient basically from the waist down. The biggest problem for me was that in order for the anesthesiologist to insert the medication, I had to first tightly curl forward, therefore exposing and emphasizing the vertebrae of my spine. I felt like I was being asked to become one of those contortionists in the circus who can curl herself into a tiny ball before being shot out of a cannon. It was nearly impossible to get my spine to arc above my belly. Both the anesthesiologist and I were not exactly having fun.

Finally I had an epiphany. If I didn't relax and talk my body into cooperating, they would have no other choice than to use a general anesthesia. I played my last "sheer will" card and my body complied. My reward was a blessed numbness—and Jon's face. He had been anxiously waiting outside the operating room for this procedure to be done.

Jon took a seat on a stool placed near my head, and I can't describe the relief I felt at his presence. Dr. Botti prepared to begin the surgery, and I said, "Wait! I want Jon to pray!" With every nerve stretched taut, the doctor wanted no more delays, but I insisted. By that point Dr. Botti knew me well enough to know that when I had my heart set on something, it was not going to be very easy to persuade me otherwise. I'm sure he weighed the time it would take to pray against the time spent arguing with me and saw the wisdom in allowing the quick prayer.

Jon's prayer echoed in the sterile room. "Father, please guide the hands of the surgeon. Allow the babies to be born healthy and for Kate to be okay." I smiled at the resounding "Amen" from so many in the room.

In what seemed like only seconds, I felt the vertical incision being made, and at 7:51 a.m. on the morning of May 10, 2004, the first of the sextuplets was born. As a squirmy tiny body emerged, Jon stated loudly for all to hear, "That's Alexis Faith!"

The entire room erupted in applause. Now that I know her, I'm not surprised it was Alexis who would feel the need to be first at the birthday party to receive a thundering applause. I am positive her heart was smiling.

• MULTIPLE BLESSINGS

As rehearsed and practiced, little Alexis weighing in at 2 lbs. 11.5 ozs. was quickly handed off to her awaiting team of neonatal doctors and nurses all sporting the letter A, for Baby A, on their scrubs. Alexis, along with her next three siblings, would be escorted by his or her own team to a second room across the hall where it was much less crowded. There each baby would be stabilized before being transported to the NICU. The last two babies, E and F, were examined and evaluated by their coinciding teams in the OR and then followed their brothers and sisters to the special care nursery.

The next three minutes were a joyful blur. As teams stood at attention awaiting their prize, I envisioned myself as a giant piñata that was torn open, dropping tiny goodies into the hands of eager participants. I was beaten and bedraggled and holding on by a thread, but by the grace of God, I was adding life to the party, literally.

Straining to see something, anything, over the blue drape blocking my limited view, I heard Jon exclaim, "Hannah Joy!" She weighed in at 2 lbs. 11 ozs. and was quickly scooped up by Team B. Baby C, our very first little boy—"Aaden Jonathan!"—was the smallest of the bunch, weighing just 2 lbs. 7.5 ozs. Seconds later Aaden became a big brother as Jon called out, "Collin Thomas!" Collin, the only one to break the three pound mark, even though it was just by a mere half an ounce, appeared to be quite a bit bigger than his "big" brother! Next came our Leah Hope with a shockingly full head of black hair and weighing 2 lbs. 14.8 ozs. And last but never least came Jon's final announcement, "Joel Kevin!" and off he went, all 2 lbs. 9.7 ozs. of him, in a bustling blur of green scrubs.

I think most mothers would agree that the several moments, or maybe hours, after giving birth, are a blur of sleepy fuzziness. Above and through it all, however, is the unquenchable thirst to see your baby. I was certainly no different. I patiently endured the stitching, the mending, and the general cleanup of an operating room that basically looked like a bomb had just hit. Jon, my oh-so-observant husband, was dutifully reporting to me on the condition of my poor overused uterus. He said it looked something like a deflated basketball as it sat sadly abandoned by the whole darn team. I didn't really see the humor in that.

Before too long I found myself back on more familiar footing: the postpartum unit on the third floor. As I settled into my room, a few family members trickled in—and best of all, Ruth arrived with Mady and Cara in tow. They had many, many questions, which I tried to patiently answer as everything within me kept screaming, "When can I see my babies?"

Hours passed as visitors came and went. I was amazed when I had a surprise visit from the infamous Joe Paterno, head coach of Penn State football. He happened to be at the hospital that day and asked if he could pop in to congratulate us. Jon shook his hand and excitedly hurried off to check in yet again on the babies and release the news to the media at 4:00 p.m.

Meanwhile I repeatedly asked anyone and everyone who passed, "Have you seen the babies? How are they?" I was practically frantic as it was approaching 8:00 p.m.—almost a full twelve hours since I had given birth, and yet I still hadn't seen even one of them for more than a split second. I was grateful for my sister Kendra who steadfastly sat by my side as people came and went, reporting what little they could to try and soothe my anxious nerves.

Finally at 9:00 p.m., my chariot arrived—a wheelchair. I was given the green light to head to the NICU to see my six premature babies I had held close to my heart for twenty-nine weeks and five days. Although in previous conversations, the nurses expressed their reservations about whether or not I would be strong enough to sit in a wheelchair to travel up four floors to see the babies on delivery day, I was determined. Weak and pale with exhaustion, I resolved myself to sit upright in that chair to get a clear view of each tiny face.

As Jon pushed me through the double doors of the high tech nursery, I looked for the names on the isolettes. They were arranged by birth order and stretched throughout the entire NICU, beginning with Alexis who greeted us at the door. There they all were, all lined up. Six teeny little veiny people. They were so adorable. Each looked like a fragile baby bird in a coiled nest of wires. I took a deep breath and slowly began my rounds. When envisioning this moment weeks before, I knew I wanted to say two important things to each baby. First, I told each baby that I loved him or her and that he or she was created for a purpose. Second, I whispered to them that I was so very sorry that they had to be there in that nursery with so many tubes and needles, monitors and machines.

I silently thanked God with all my heart for sending those doctors and nurses, angels on earth, to care for my babies with such gentle and wise expertise.

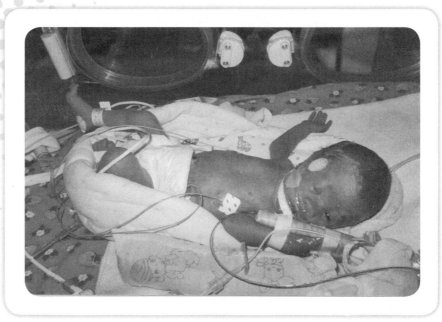

Alexis Faith

8 Our Fragile but Feisty Fighters

For you formed my inward parts;
   You covered me in my mother's womb.
I will praise You, for I am fearfully and
   wonderfully made.

Psalm 139:13 – 14 NKJV

I was discharged from the hospital on Friday, May 15, five days after the birth of the babies. I was still reeling from my ever-changing hormone levels, and physically I felt weak and depleted. Having been on bed rest for so long, I had lost significant muscle mass in my lower body and walking left me shaky and exhausted. Also, after all those days confined to the four walls of my room longing to be outside, and better yet, to be home, I suddenly found myself not at all ready to leave the protective and steady routine of the hospital. But I had no choice. My insurance company had decided it was time for me to go home.

Looking out the window on that last day as I sat waiting for Jon, I thought back to a few days prior to my discharge when Jon had wheeled me outside for the very first time. It was so completely overwhelming. I felt like a momma bear who had gone into hibernation only to awaken to a whole new fresh and fragrant spring.

Jon was amazed as I sat there and just sobbed. Those who know anything about me know this: I am definitely not a nature girl. But on that day I just couldn't get enough. It was as if the grass was suddenly greener, the sky was clearer, and the flowers were sweeter. The world was like a beautiful kaleidoscope of color and it was almost too much for me to take in. Just the sound of the birds singing to each other in the tree above my head stirred up a deep appreciation for nature that I hadn't been aware of before. I decided that day that I would never again take God's gifts of the great outdoors for granted, even if I am just the type to admire it from afar.

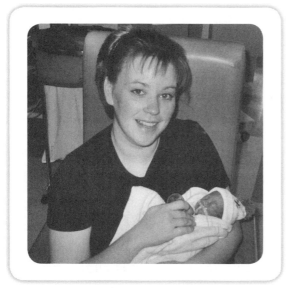

Hannah Joy (with Mommy)

That day made me realize all that I had missed during my time in the hospital, and I feared that I would be expected to just pick up where I left off with no allowance for culture shock.

Even worse than the fear of being expected to just jump right back into my old life, was the overwhelming sadness at leaving my precious babies behind. It is one of the most unnatural things a mother can be asked to do. How was I expected to actually go down the elevator, out the door, and into a waiting car that would drive away from six parts of my very own heart? As I went through the NICU to say good-bye that day, I felt my heart breaking and six pieces drop with a heavy thud right there on the cold sterile floor as I quietly wheeled by each incubator whispering promises of my quick return.

As I left the hospital, I convinced Jon that maybe it would lift our spirits to stop at the grocery store and pick up the ingredients for a celebration dinner. I missed cooking, and I was desperate to do something that felt normal. So off to the grocery store we went — only to realize that a stroll around the aisles was more than a bit ambitious for my first day out. We grabbed the ingredients for filet mignon with teriyaki sauce, asparagus, and grilled potatoes, a favorite for both of us that was reserved for very special occasions. We hopped, well more like hobbled, into the car and started off for my parents' house where we were to stay so we could be close to the babies.

We weren't very far down the road when I discovered we had a problem: my "bladder" was full. I still had a Foley catheter, which is an indwelling catheter with a clear plastic bag attached to collect urine, and there was no way we could drive another mile without stopping to empty it. Gross as it sounds, we had no choice other than to pull over on the side of the road for a pit stop. Having spent every ounce of energy on my grocery store expedition I found it wonderfully convenient to just point the darn tube out the door and, well, go. Jon and I laughed uncontrollably with tears streaming down our faces as we sat listening to the incessant ppssssst as the bag emptied. We would gain control for a minute only to glance at each other and once again gasp breathlessly as the pent up stress tumbled out in fits of uproarious laughter.

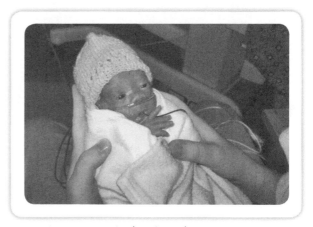

Aaden Jonathan

When we finally arrived at my parents' house with months of my acquired belongings to unload from the car, my mom wondered aloud what in the world had taken us so long. We managed to piece together the story through still stifled giggles like two teenagers trying to explain why they were late for curfew. It was one of those you-had-to-be-there moments, and my mom just shooed us into the house. To my relief, she had already prepared a nice dinner of chicken and mashed potatoes.

Dinner, however, didn't turn out to be the celebration Jon and I had envisioned. It was instead upsetting for my girls. Their young world was about to be rocked yet again with another big change, and they were feeling every not-so-subtle hint. Mady and Cara basically misbehaved to the point of tears—for both them and me.

The thought crossed my brain that "I guess I should just go back." Obviously I knew I couldn't go back—and I didn't want to go back—but I couldn't deny that going forward was difficult. How could I possibly explain all of that to two very confused three-year-olds? It broke my heart because I knew exactly what was happening; they were wondering who was now in charge. As they tested the waters, I tried my best to be patient and understanding. I knew the girls had been forced to adapt to many changes, and my reappearance had just sent them over the edge.

●

As each day passed, we would go to visit the babies in the NICU. It became a familiar and almost strangely soothing place, with all its bells and beepers constantly monitoring the details of each baby's delicate condition. We felt blessed that six state-of-the-art incubators, called Giraffe isolettes, a gift to the hospital from the Children's Miracle Network, were reserved for my babies. The beds provided warmth under a special memory foam mattress and were made with a top that could be raised or lowered, allowing the physicians to effectively control the environment that each individual baby required. Expert and loving care was showered on the babies as they slowly learned to breathe, suck, swallow, and even grow.

Meanwhile, I was falling more in love each day as I noted their subtle differences—like Collin's full and rosy lips and Leah's delicate little China-doll face. Once again I was humbled at the expanse of God's creation and grace as I sat on those early spring mornings watching new life tentatively erupt outside the window while my babies' budding personalities unfurled inside the nursery. Like the tiniest seedlings peeking their heads through the cold hard ground, they were so very small and fragile and yet possessed a strength and tenacity that made me as proud as the mother of any hulking NFL player.

Jon and I cheered our babies on as they gained a half ounce here and a half ounce there. We were awed each day to see the distinct features of each baby revealed as they gradually grew a bit more infantlike. Leah's hair instantly identified her, so dark and silky black. Hannah was her closest look-alike, and together they managed to instantly wind some nurses' heartstrings around their teensy little fingers. It was difficult at times to tell one from the other.

Alexis was lighter skinned than her two sisters, her hair was blonde, and her face was rounder. She had spunk and an inner charisma that somehow translated into "Look out world, here I come!"

Collin was easy to pick out of the crowd. He was really only a few ounces bigger than the others during most stretches of time,

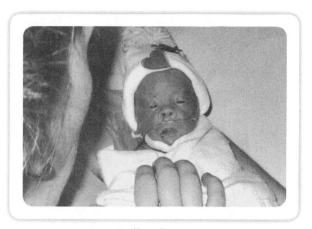

Collin Thomas

but it was noticeable, especially because his head was bigger. He was the slowest to develop, struggling to breathe on his own for quite a few weeks after the others were weaned from CPAP. (Fortunately Collin has not only grown into his head but has developed an equally big heart and smile to match.)

Aaden was a ringer for Jon's dad, although—I hate to say it—my very first thought was, "Oh my goodness! He looks like a tiny bald squirrel." We all know I meant that in the most loving motherly way! He was after all, the smallest of the group, and the only one without hair. (Sorry, Aaden! But don't worry, your cuteness quotient skyrocketed as soon as you reached five pounds!)

Joel was just a tad darker skinned than Aaden and much more laid back. The very first time I laid eyes on Joel I gasped loudly. There in front of my eyes was a miniature sleeping Jon; his mouth, his eyes, his expression—everything. I didn't know then that Joel, who was already considered by the nursing staff to be the "quiet little guy in the back row who just minded his own business," would grow into an exact replica of his daddy's personality—not too many ups, not too many downs, just steady and relaxed, go with the flow, and never in a hurry.

Mady and Cara were busy growing in their own way during those hectic weeks. They were very used to hearing hospital jargon by that time, and at three years old they used words like *NICU, preemies, CPAP,* and *sextuplets* as a normal part of their pretend play. I'm not sure they

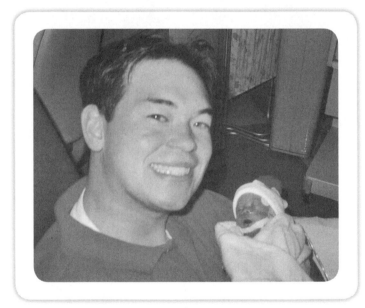

Leah Hope (and Daddy)

really thought anything unusual about their brothers and sisters, neither the number of them or the miniature size of them. The twins were spared all of the sleepless nights filled with worry about whether Aaden was over stimulated by an IV change or if Leah had spit up her entire feeding.

They spent many of those afternoons with my mom while I went to the hospital to pace around the room of specialized incubators. When the girls occasionally got to tag along, they were usually clutching their newest friends, two stuffed animals given to them by a friend. To this day Mady has Tubby, a floppy green hippo, and Cara sleeps with Slumber, a beloved brown bear. These two longtime buddies have been through it all with the twins, and are now irreplaceable.

My days fell into a somewhat disheveled routine. I, not surprisingly, found it difficult to be at the mercy of others when I knew what I had in my mind to do. It took excruciating patience for all of us as my mom and dad tried to weave the many loose threads of my life into their once peaceful daily schedule. I had one thing and only one thing on my mind during every waking moment: finish what needs to be tended to—whether it was a shower for me, a meal for the girls, or other daily chores—so I could get to the NICU to see my babies. It seemed like an eternity before my mom and I could finally set off for the short ride to the hospital each afternoon. She would drop me off and later come back to pick me up. Still unable to sit for a very long time, I only lasted about forty-five minutes at first, but later thankfully was able to stay about two to four hours, and eventually the entire day.

When I would walk through the doors of the NICU after having scrubbed my hands and arms carefully, I would always try to quickly assess the mood of the room. Was it a stressful day with doctors and nurses huddling over beeping monitors or was it instead a day when I was instantly greeted with an "everything's been fine" kind of smile? I would usually get a blow-by-blow description from the attending nurses on how each baby had done throughout the night, who was "behaving," and who was stirring up some trouble that day. During the report, somewhere around baby number three, I would have to remind myself to breathe because I was always fearful that we would make it through the first few and maybe at the end, I would have some bad news. I praise God that there were very few times I had any real reason to worry.

My special treat on any given day was the opportunity to actually pick up and hold one or more of my babies. I had held Hannah on the day I left the hospital. She was five days old but stable enough to breathe with only the help of CPAP and could tolerate touch. Jon and

I, on the other hand, could hardly find our breath. She was merely a sweet mushy center in a bundle of soft blankets. I remember leaning in to gently kiss her little forehead. My lips were actually bigger than her crinkled tiny brow, and it felt like I had just kissed her whole face.

I am going to admit something here that I have received much criticism for: I wholeheartedly bonded with Hannah that day, the first of my babies that I could actually hold and snuggle. She and I sort of grew this unexplainable instant attachment from the start. She seemed to respond to me as I did to her, and we mutually fed each other's need to nurture and be nurtured. I am not saying that I did not bond with my other children; I am simply saying for the sole benefit of the other mothers of multiples out there, that we are human. It is, I believe, quite natural to bond more easily with a baby whom you have held and snuggled.

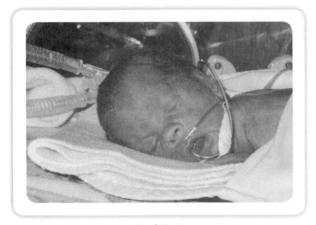

Joel Kevin

Poor Collin struggled for two whole weeks to finally get to the point where I could do anything more than reach into his isolette and stroke his little arm or leg. I feel that consequently Collin and I did not properly bond until months later. But I am stating for the record and for the world to know, I, like any mother of more than one child, love my children differently but equally. And the relationships with our children grow and change. Now, three and a half years later, Collin is affectionately known by all as "Mommy's helper boy!" I have no question at all whether he knows he is loved wholeheartedly.

One morning I wheeled up to the NICU counter in my wheelchair, feeling awful—awful that my babies were being poked and prodded, that they were straining to learn the crash course of breathing and eating. I was immensely disappointed in myself because I hadn't been able to hold out for them any longer. Just a few more days of being pregnant would've given them more strength for the fight for their lives. I felt guilty and miserable.

Dr. Mujsce came over to me as he was doing his rounds. Being a man surrounded by emotional mothers every single day, he immediately read my palpable sadness. Without hesitation he looked me in the eye and told me a story. After the birth of the sextuplets, a world renowned placenta pathologist came to the hospital to study the half dozen placentas for scientific research. What he found was astounding. Dr. Mujsce kindly recited three main points: First, my placentas were the healthiest the pathologist had ever seen. Second, they were "strategically placed for optimum growth." Third, the pathologist felt that I had "delivered at the top of the mountain." In other words, just a few more days and the health of one or more of the babies could have been severely compromised. With finality in his voice Dr. Mujsce kindly yet firmly told me it was time to "hang up my disappointment."

I felt immense relief wash over me. I thanked God for using the babies' doctor that day to reveal those details so I could commit my energy and focus to the miraculous minute-by-minute milestones they were reaching every day.

While emotions ran high in the nursery, life at home was also wrought with stress. We were still staying at my parents' house, and I longed to regain ownership of my days, my girls, and my life. I wanted to be "Mommy" again. I hated feeling that they had somehow drifted away from me, and like a mother hen wanting to collect her chicks, I wanted them under my wing, if not under my roof. Jon saw my need and he made a phone call to the social worker in the NICU explaining our situation.

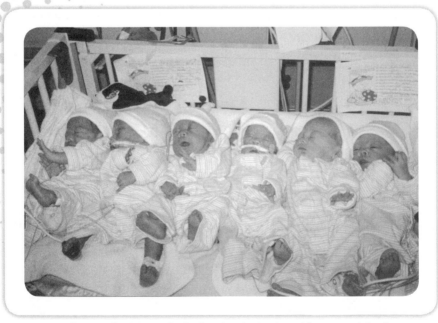

*Left to right: Hannah, Collin, Leah, Aaden, Alexis, and Joel
on the day we brought Hannah and Leah home: June 26, 2004.*

9 Displaced, Together

He who fears the LORD has a secure fortress,
and for his children it will be a refuge.

Proverbs 14:26

By the grace of God and the diligence of the social worker, we were told we could move into the Ronald McDonald House in Hershey, Pennsylvania, just minutes from the hospital. The house contains twenty-five bedrooms and offers a refuge to the families of seriously ill children. Tentatively walking into the open and well-appointed kitchen where several families gathered for meals, I was awed. It was any woman's dream kitchen, yet I clutched Mady's and Cara's hands tightly as I realized this would be a learning experience for me. Being severely "germophobic" I was leery of sharing plates, utensils, and appliances with complete strangers.

That initial discomfort was short-lived. I was truly "Mommy" for the first time in over six months, and Jon and I were so blissfully happy to reclaim our family foursome. I felt as if I had just escaped some sort of weird time warp, and everyday mundane things became a rite of passage back into motherhood. It would take almost a full two hours for me to shower, pump breast milk for the babies, get the girls dressed, and feed the girls each a bowl of cereal, but I was thrilled to actively be back in the game of life.

Initially, I would pack the girls a lunch and we would drop them both off at my brother and sister-in law's house to play while we went to the hospital. Occasionally a friend, Suzanne, would also offer to keep them. Eventually, I met a family who was also staying at the Ronald McDonald House while their infant son recovered in the NICU. In fact, he was Aaden's neighbor. The family, who had an older son around the same age as the girls, was from an area near our hometown

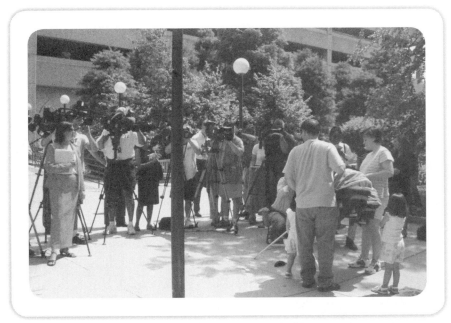

Hannah and Leah going home surrounded by a media storm.

and we instantly hit it off. Amy and I shared similar mothering styles and soon came to the conclusion that we could help one another by trading babysitting duties throughout the day. The girls were thrilled to have a new friend and I was thankful that the arrangement worked very well for both of us. I was very conscious of not exhausting my family members and friends with more requests for babysitting after they had already been helping me for months.

News spread of our large family, and Jon and I were invited to be the recipients of a home makeover presented as a gift from a new television show. Jon and I drove home to our little three-bedroom house to meet the film crew there, and I was so nervous. I had not been home in so long that it felt surreal as we pulled into the driveway. I asked myself, "Could it really have been just a few months?" Everything in our life had changed so drastically that our house felt like an old friend I hadn't seen in a long time—familiar yet awkward. We arrived in the late evening and slept well. Soon the film crew arrived to document our thoughts as we walked through our home, discussing aloud the different changes that were being proposed.

I should have been ecstatic at this answer to prayer. Never did I think we would have so much help in trying to reconfigure our house so that all of us could live more comfortably. However, I was a wreck. I had woken up that morning and decided to retrieve my cell phone messages. I was not overly attached to my cell phone and I seldom remembered to regularly check my calls. When I heard the doctor's voice and noticed the message was left in the wee hours of the morning, my heart skipped a beat. Adding a whole new twist to an already stressful day, we learned our little Aaden was experiencing what is known as A's and B's, apnea's and bradycardias. Apneas meant he would stop breathing for seconds at a time, which consequently resulted in bradycardias, a drop in his heart rate. The even bigger scare was the question of whether or not he was developing a condition called necrotizing enterocolitis, which is an infection in the intestinal tract that can be serious enough that the intestinal tract begins to die off. Obviously it could potentially be an extremely threatening situation and we were told that Aaden had been immediately sent for bowel X-rays. He would be given antibiotics and his tube feedings would stop.

I stood rooted to one spot in my kitchen clutching the phone close to my ear, desperate to not lose one detail of the information being given to me. As a nurse I fully understood the situation and the potential implications. At that moment, with cameras on me and people waiting for my participation, I felt panic creeping in. All that mattered was Aaden and he was an hour away. I didn't care about paint, dishwashers, decorative touches, or social etiquette for that matter. I just wanted to get to my baby.

However, I was intimidated by the seeming importance of the official visit from a television crew and I didn't have the gumption to say, "Sorry for the inconvenience, guys, but I'm out of here!" I spent all day feigning interest while praying feverishly that it would all end soon so I could go to be with my son.

When I couldn't take it one more minute, I looked at Jon, pleading with my eyes for him to understand. Thankfully, he knows me well and said, "Kate, just go." That was all I needed. I was out that front door in two minutes, knowing Jon was capable of handling whatever still needed to be discussed. I drove like a madwoman on twisting back roads through a blinding rainstorm. I felt like I was in a movie with a suspenseful plot. Could it possibly get any worse, I wondered?

When I finally arrived at the NICU frazzled and fearful, I hurried over to Aaden's incubator. He was being tended to by a traveling male nurse I had never seen before. When I asked if I could hold Aaden, I was told that he had had a very rough day and that no, holding him would not be permitted at the moment. I knew my son needed me, yet I couldn't even touch him.

I tried to remain calm, reassuring myself that he was getting the best care possible. I figured I would allow the nurse to do his work without me hovering nervously over him, and so I slowly made my way around the room to see my five other babies. After visiting with each of them, I returned to Aaden in hopes that he had settled down enough to be taken out of the incubator. I found him resting peacefully, his little face showing no sign of the turmoil of the day. Not wanting to disturb him, I quietly studied his delicate features and thanked God my little guy had such tenacity and strength. I promised myself that day that I would never again allow anything or anyone to come before my kids. Sometimes I might step on toes, wound some egos, or seem like I am asking too much, but my number one priority after my God and my husband will always be my eight children.

The blessings kept pouring in. Within just two weeks of moving into the Ronald McDonald House we received the news that through the generosity of the Hershey Corporation, we would be allowed the use of a beautiful condo-minium. We would be welcome to reside there right up until that won-derful day when all ten of us would finally make the hour-long drive to our own home. It was the first time in so very, very long that we could actually be alone. It's amazing how much I took something as abstract as privacy for granted until it became nonexistent in my life.

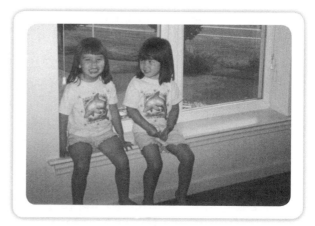

Cara and Mady's favorite spot in the condo: the windowsill.

At the memory of our previous attempt to make a celebratory din-ner we decided that this time a frozen pizza with only the four of us would be just fine. So on our first night in the condo, June 11, one day before our fifth wedding anniversary, we sat enjoying our quick meal while once again marveling at the generosity of people who didn't even know us. We felt immensely blessed and asked ourselves for maybe the millionth time, "Is this really all happening or are we going to wake up to find it was all just a dream?"

The condo was sheer bliss. It had a living room with a pull-out couch, a large television, a master bedroom with a king-sized bed, a kitchen, a dining room, and an additional bedroom with two double beds. We were giddy at the thought of being able to finally spread out and we quickly got busy making it a place where we could feel at home and comfortable.

The first thing Jon did was to set up a "pumping station" near a big overstuffed chair in the bedroom. The sight of that calm little corner of the world brought tears to my eyes. My favorite part was that it was positioned perfectly by the window to allow me a bird's eye view of the pool outside. On sunny days I would sit and watch Jon splashing and laughing with the girls in the water. I spent many hours in the chair, attempting to pump enough milk to supply each baby's bottle at every feeding. A short time later, however, I learned an important lesson in mothering higher order multiples: a few ounces of breast milk carefully divvied up six ways was really not going to offer the same benefit that a good solid full feeding could offer the two weakest babies, Collin and Aaden. I learned that being the mother of six infants I was going to need to tend to the most critical problems first; from that point on, Collin and Aaden received most, if not all, of my "liquid gold."

I took this "milk lesson" to heart, knowing that I, just like the milk, could easily be of little good to anyone if I spread myself too thin. I was most helpful if I gave my full attention to whoever needed me the most at any given time.

The second lesson I learned during our stay at the condo was that we actually needed surprisingly little to survive. The four of us had spent more than a month with just a few changes of clothes and several packed boxes courtesy of the Ronald McDonald House. The gracious volunteers at the Ronald McDonald House had ushered me to the basement on the day we moved out. There on meticulously organized shelves was tons of food and dry goods, and I was told "Help yourself. Take anything you need." I stood in wonder as once again God had met all of our needs and beyond. Also, I felt humbled to my core at the willingness of people to open their heart, their home, and now their pantry to help care for my family. They had become another piece in the large puzzle God was constructing to demonstrate to us His vision and grace.

These lessons, along with all those learned throughout my pregnancy, began a huge transition in my heart and my life. In my earlier days of motherhood with the twins, I confess I had a fond attachment to material things. My two girls were always impeccably dressed with just the right matching hair ribbon and of course the perfect shoes to complete their ensemble. I drew a direct connection between two clean, well-dressed kids and my success as a mother. My drive was not powered by greed or narcissism; I simply felt compelled to be, look, and do the best that I possibly could in all things and in all ways. That high ambition sometimes spilled over into discontent and impossible-to-meet demands. That aspect of my personality has been a thorn in my side, and to this day I often need to remind myself of how very little we had during those months at the Hershey condo and yet how completely happy we were because we had each other and we had our eight healthy kids.

From the moment I discovered I was pregnant with sextuplets, God took me to a place of utter dependency on Him—financially, physically, emotionally, psychologically. As I learned to lean on Him and trust Him completely, God, because of His goodness and grace, blessed me with more than I could've ever hoped or imagined: more children, more joy, more faith, and—okay, even more laundry. Now I can stand over my mountains of laundry and actually be thankful. I thank God every day that I have children to wear the clothes, and clothes to dress the children.

Although we spent only a total of five weeks at our haven in the condo, daily life was rapidly changing. Every day the babies were growing, getting stronger and healthier. Tests were routinely performed to assure they were developing on par—CAT scans checking for brain bleeds, a common complication in preemies; heart valves that needed to close on their own; eye development, another common concern with babies who are so small. As always Jon and I breathed a sigh of relief as each and every test on every single baby came back with great results. Dr. Mujsce commented several times that having six out of six infants be 100 percent healthy was an absolute miracle. We wholeheartedly agreed.

We began to look forward to the day that the doctors would eventually begin to release each of them from the hospital. As exciting as that was, it was also nerve-wracking. What in the world did we really know about being solely responsible for six high-risk premature infants? How could anyone truly be prepared anyway? Our lives had been a series of one unpredictable event after another for so long, I couldn't imagine the energy, organization, and flexibility it was going to take to somehow regain our stability as a couple and as a family.

On the other hand, I began to feel a familiar nesting instinct kick in. Realizing the babies would be at significant risk of sickness and infection, we set about making the environment in the condo as germ-free and safe as possible for them. First, Jon shampooed the carpets. We then moved the dining room furniture out of the way to allow for more floor space for pack and plays and I draped each couch in fresh white cotton sheets, attempting to decrease any pollutants and dust that might be a problem.

Cara and Mady felt the impending excitement as well but were much more engrossed in the train that regularly passed maybe a hundred yards from their bedroom window. They would perch on a wide windowsill in anticipation of the bone-rattling roar of the passing train. Once Jon discovered Cara in the middle of the night snuggled up on the windowsill, clutching her buddy Slumber, having fallen asleep there in the middle of her watch.

I was proud of Mady and Cara for adjusting to their latest home, but I still felt like I needed the peace of mind of knowing that they would get the attention they deserved when the babies finally arrived. Therefore, after learning that Hannah and Leah would be the first babies to be discharged, it was decided that the girls would make their first overnight voyage to Jon's mom's house on the day after their sisters' discharge. With my days still consumed by so many unknowns, it was a great relief to know that the girls would be safe and sound with Grandmom, being loved and entertained.

I realized that even with all my careful preparation, I hadn't thought of what the babies would wear to come home from the hospital. That's when Amy, the friend I had met at the Ronald McDonald House, happened to show me a sweet little dress that she had been given when she was expecting. As we oohed and aahed over her baby boy who would obviously not need the dress, she asked if I would want it. It was creamy white, wonderfully girly, and covered in sweet purple flowers. Not only was it adorable, it also had a cute floppy hat to match. It was absolutely perfect, and since it had been recently purchased we thought we might be able to find two more so all three baby girls could be dressed alike. Later that day, Jon and I did indeed make a trip to Babies "R" Us and easily found the other dresses! We also made our first boy purchases, three pale blue linen outfits with sailor type hats. I was so excited to see how handsome our three little guys would look in their first official clothes.

On June 26, we left the hospital with six-week-old Hannah Joy and Leah Hope. As we went through the doors we were greeted by a rather large group of news reporters and photographers. It was still very overwhelming for me as I felt protective of my two little girls who could barely be seen above the sides of their car seats. Everyone jockeyed for position, and flashbulbs went off as we made our way out to our waiting car. We were on such an emotional high that we felt we were walking on air. It was difficult to absorb just how far we had come and that we were one giant step further along our long, long road to getting our family home.

As we opened the door to our condo we were greeted with six brand new compact, easy to store pack and play cribs. Jon and I looked from one to the other, wondering how in the world they had gotten there. We were soon informed that employees from Babies "R" Us had gotten permission to sneak into our borrowed space and set up the pack and plays as a welcome "home" surprise. It was a very practical and valuable surprise because neither of us had a real plan as far as sleeping arrangements for the babies went. It seems silly to not know such a huge detail. The pack and plays were well used from that day forward for probably close to three years when the babies finally grew too long to take even a quick nap in them at a friend's house.

The next morning we kissed Cara and Madelyn good-bye as they set off for their exciting adventure to Grandmom's house. We had not set a specific length of time for their stay as we did not know what the next few days would involve in regard to more babies being released from the hospital. We agreed that they would stay with their grandmother until they showed signs of homesickness and had had enough, probably a week. Jon's mom was wonderful as she chattered happily about all the big girl things she had planned for their visit. I gave a sigh of relief as curiosity and wonder sparkled in Mady's and Cara's brown eyes as they gave me one last big hug before grabbing Grandmom's hand and leaving the four of us behind.

It was odd for the first few hours: Jon and I had a major sense of déjà vu with our two baby girls. It was suddenly uncharacteristically quiet in the condo, and we decided to put Hannah and Leah into Mady and Cara's old double stroller and go outside for a walk in the fresh air. As we walked together on a beautiful warm early summer afternoon, we felt content and under control. "Didn't we just do this three years ago?" we marveled. We knew twins, we knew girls—we had done this part before. Buoyed by the energetic and maybe naïve confidence of youth, we walked with a new bounce in our step, putting out of our minds for just one afternoon the fact that four more little people would soon arrive to forever redefine our definition of "under control."

It wasn't very long before I was asking Dr. Mujsce when he would be giving me more babies. I believe my words to him were, "Bring it on!" He just smiled in his calm doctor-ish way and said he didn't want us to get overwhelmed but, "Soon."

He kept his word, and on Wednesday, June 30, Jon and I once again dressed Hannah and Leah in their beautiful little matching dresses to go pick up their sister Alexis. "Triplets. We can do this," we thought. And we did. In spite of the fact that we were growing more and more exhausted, we were still able to think coherently and we began to devise a more concrete workable schedule.

Ironically, Jon was able to take an active role in helping to set that foundation only because he had been unceremoniously let go from his job for the second time since we learned I was pregnant. It happened a few days before we brought Hannah and Leah home. He had been working for a petroleum company, and after fixing their network and later handing in his insurance information, having worked there for just one month, he was told that he was no longer needed.

The first time Jon lost his job, it was difficult. Not only was the timing horrible with me being pregnant at the time, but it obviously was demoralizing in practically every respect. If we thought the first time had been tough, the second time was pure torture. Suddenly fear set in with a vengeance. What if this pattern continued and basically destroyed any chance of Jon being able to provide for our family? Would anybody be willing to hire Jon ever again? How in the world would we feed, clothe, and house our children? I had no idea sometimes where we would be in a week and if I allowed my thoughts to wander too far ahead; it physically made me sick.

As doubt and uncertainty reared their ugly heads, one silver lining could be found in the large and gloomy storm cloud hovering over our heads. Jon had the opportunity to help me with the transition of bringing the babies home. He was there to help with feeding, changing, and bathing our babies, which probably was the sole reason I survived, we survived. I realized much, much later with the wisdom that only hindsight can offer that I would've never been able to handle the physical and emotional demands of taking care of the babies by myself at that time. Also, I imagine it would've been difficult to stay connected as a couple if he left each morning for his corporate world while I was left behind at home drowning in a sea of bottles, diapers, and demanding cries.

Joel was the next baby to be released from the hospital — the first of the three boys. By that time our days in the condo with the three girls were much more challenging, so we decided it would make sense for Jon to stay home with them while I went to pick up our son. Joel's coming home picture taken on July 2 was drastically different than that of his sisters. It was just tiny little Joel in his car seat. No major newspaper photographers, reporters, or other media were waiting. I hadn't even bathed him before dressing him; for me, that was one small example of how my need for control was loosening. Honestly, Joel's homecoming was the best of them all — a tender memory for me as I think of our peaceful ride home. Had I known that it would be the only time Joel and I would have alone for maybe the whole first year of his life, I would've valued those fifteen minutes even more.

Joel was not an easy baby on his first few days at the condo. He was generally unsettled and had a nearly constant low pitch whine. We would jiggle, sway, rock, and walk him, but it wasn't until my sister Chris arrived that we, or rather she, found the magic touch. She somehow always managed to get him settled down. We had asked Chris to come when we realized that we needed a night feeder. She was a great sport even though she was twenty weeks pregnant herself. She readily packed up Meghan, her seven-year-old daughter, and came from Ohio to lend an extra pair of hands for almost a week and a half.

Thanks to Chris and her seemingly endless supply of energy, we managed quite nicely with the four babies who were home. Although each day was somewhat of a blur, Jon and I still managed to go to the hospital daily to check in on Collin and Aaden. Collin was still the biggest baby but was just physically weaker and less reactive. He was taking his own sweet time in maturing to the point where he could be discharged. Aaden, on the other hand, had been born the smallest, but developmentally, he had always been on the same time frame as the girls. However, when he suffered the frightening setback, he fell way behind and it took him several weeks to fully recover.

Right about the time Aunt Chris had to leave, it was finally time for Collin and Aaden to join the clan at the condo. I stopped Chris at the door right before she left and made her demonstrate her "magic touch" that she used on Joel. It was the first time in my adult life that I could picture myself falling on the floor and grasping someone's ankles to prevent her from leaving.

She saw and fully understood my desperation, but gave her good-natured laugh as she demonstrated a quick tutorial in her well-rehearsed Joel sway. It felt so odd for me to actually have to ask someone what made my own baby happy. I hated that I had not had the time to figure it out myself. With dividing myself four ways, I simply couldn't be present long enough to pick up on Joel's quirks. That bothered me, and I soon realized that it was just the tip of the iceberg. Many, many times in the weeks and months to come I would need to defer to other people to feed, snuggle, calm, and rock my children. I did not easily learn or accept this piece of my reality.

On July 9, Aaden weighed nearly five pounds and was sent home with a monitor to warn us if he should stop breathing at any time. Hannah had also been sent home with a monitor, and having been around the buzzing and beeping for two months by that time, it didn't seem so scary. It was actually fairly routine for premature babies to "forget" to breathe at times. Their systems were still playing catch-up, and sometimes it was as if they would just go on overload.

Collin was a hefty six and a half pounds when he left the hospital with his brother that day. He actually looked like he had some roundness to his cheeks as I happily tucked him in his car seat for the ride home to the condo. I couldn't believe as I drove out of the long and winding driveway of the hospital that I would have all six of my babies with me in one place. I was exhausted, exhilarated, excited, and I guess in a way, exonerated. I think many people thought I was a bit crazy throughout my pregnancy, with things like demanding my vitamins, getting weekly massages, singing until I went hoarse in my attempt to stay positive, and believing in my God. However, as

I walked out of that hospital with the last of my six healthy babies, I believe more than a few were awed by the miracle they had watched unfold.

●

Later that night when Jon and I collapsed into bed, we laid there in the darkness of our bedroom surrounded by three pack and plays, each containing two tightly swaddled infants. Aaah! Quiet. But not for long. All around us were soft snorty little grunts and snores. In a tired, perplexed voice Jon asked, "Do we have goats?" That was enough to set off a serious case of sleep deprivation giggles. We laughed for almost a full hour, as each time we would settle down, we would hear another little nasal noise and start laughing all over again. It felt good to laugh, to have joy fill the room as finally we had our miracle babies all sleeping under one roof.

By the next morning the euphoria had worn off and we looked at each other with bleary-eyed seriousness. After a long night we realized that we needed help — and fast. It had been downright scary throughout the night to go from one baby to the next, and the next, and the next, and the — well you get the idea. It seemed neverending. Just as we would each get one baby changed, fed, and back to sleep, we would quickly tend to the next in line, who was usually working himself up into a frantic squawk by that time. As daylight dawned, we felt like someone had put us on a treadmill without showing us how to stop the dumb thing. We were running and running, and yet as we raced to make bottles, give feedings, and change diapers, we felt as though we were getting nowhere fast.

Our insurance company referred us to a private nursing company that would be able to provide us with two night nurses between the hours of 11:00 p.m. and 7:00 a.m. We were desperate, and yet it was difficult to hand our high-risk preemies, two of them still wearing monitors, to complete strangers. I felt sad but knew that I needed to do what was best for the babies.

Unfortunately I had to ask myself over and over again if indeed our decision to hire outside nurses was in fact, best for the babies. The first nurses who were sent were not skilled specifically in the field of pediatrics, and especially not in dealing with babies fresh from the NICU. One particular incident confirmed all my concerns. While Jon changed Alexis's tiny diaper one morning, I heard him screaming for me. When I got to the side of the changing table, what I saw horrified me. There in Alexis's diaper was a quarter-sized chunk of a candy bar that had obviously been dropped by the visiting nurse during a hurried and haphazard middle of the night change.

I was infuriated and yet helpless. We were desperate and knew we needed help; I couldn't afford to just fire the nurses. While still trying to calm down, I made an emotionally charged phone call to the director of the nursing agency, firmly requesting that she send me the absolute best nurses on her staff. My babies and I had been through the fight of our lives and I felt they deserved white glove treatment.

I knew I once again might be criticized for such high demands, but why would I settle for less than what any mother would expect? Should my concern be watered down because my unique situation put a strain on the system? No. My concern was multiplied by six and so therefore, yes, I sometimes came across as excessively demanding. Let's face it: my life at that time was excessively demanding and my choice was to either rally to meet those demands or be swallowed up by the weighty wave of responsibility. Sinking was not something I would allow with six babies counting on me, so I unapologetically made up my mind that I would continue to do whatever it took to give my babies the loving care and attention they deserved.

New nurses were assigned, but Jon never did get to truly rest as he took it upon himself to sort of sleep with one eye open so he could monitor the care of our babies throughout the night. He is a good daddy!

The babies were on a feeding schedule of 8:00, 12:00, 4:00, and 8:00. Because they were premature, they were still slow and deliberate bottle suckers with sensitive digestive systems. It took almost a full hour at times to coax a sleepy baby to consume just three ounces of formula. By the time a baby was burped, changed, and nestled back to sleep, it was nearly time to begin heating bottles for the next feeding.

Jon and I thought we would have to grow extra arms, but thankfully help arrived. Before long, we found our condo—that at first seemed so roomy and spacious—to be a busy hub of arriving and departing volunteers. Out of a group of maybe thirty people we would somehow piece together enough helpers for each and every feeding. The job was getting done, but we quickly realized that we needed a more concrete volunteer schedule to eliminate the chances of having perhaps seven people show up for one feeding and only two show up for the next. I was unsettled knowing that one or more crying babies would need to wait if there weren't enough hands.

It seems odd that after explaining how much of a control freak I was that I didn't have a preset plan all ready to set into motion. I can only say that it was the grace of God. He knew I could take only so much at any given moment. While I was in the hospital with so much time to fret and worry, I somehow managed to have peace about the necessary help falling into place when the time was right. Matthew 6:34 says, "Therefore do not worry about tomorrow, for tomorrow will worry about itself. Each day has enough trouble of its own." Suffice it to say that each of my days definitely had enough of its own trouble; therefore I had no choice really but to trust and believe.

That is not to say that Jon and I just sat back and assumed people would jump in and help us care for

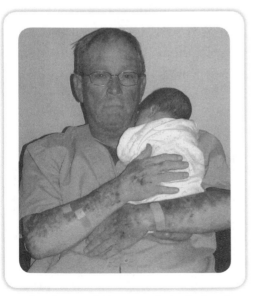

Our Poppy helping with the babies!

our hungry babies. We definitely discussed the daily challenges that would be our sole responsibility, and we brainstormed often about different possible scenarios. What I am saying is that I, the complete planner and obsessive controller that I was, had finally, finally, absorbed the fact that I could trust God to see to all the details.

My friend Marsha whom I had known since high school had been one of the people to show up at the condo to feed babies during that time. Being a natural organizer, she could see the stress of our patchwork volunteer dilemma and offered to step in and make a "real" schedule. Oh, relief! I was comforted to know I could look at the list and know that for the 4:00 p.m. feeding I would have just the right number of volunteers.

One huge frustration however was that although it was wonderful so many people wanted to help, there seemed to be just as many curious onlookers who were merely interested in seeing the babies. There were also a few who just weren't prepared for the weightless fragility of a baby that small; they seemed uncomfortable, nervous, and desperate to get out of there. The beeping monitors stressed some people out to the point of jumping every time one would go off.

Often, after Jon or I would take the time to carefully instruct a volunteer how to hold a premature infant while feeding, we would never see that person again. A few hours later, in would walk a whole new set of volunteers, most of whom had never held or fed a preemie. Once again, either Jon or I would carefully demonstrate how to hold the baby upright with his head tilted slightly back. We would explain the importance of moving the baby slowly and keeping him upright for at least a half hour after feeding to discourage an upset belly. The litany of instructions for each new volunteer grew somewhat redundant and draining in a very short time.

One afternoon, the skies were turning a horrible angry gray. The air was oppressively hot and stagnant and seemed to carry an ominous warning. Jon was just getting ready to go to Ephrata to meet my sister Kendra for an infant CPR class. He had taken it upon himself to sign up for the class, feeling that even though I was a nurse and obviously knew infant CPR, he, too, should have that knowledge. I completely agreed and was glad he thought of it, but with the skies growing dark as night in the middle of a summer afternoon, I was more than a little scared to have him leave. I begged him to stay home and take the class another day. He was not having it, and truthfully I think he had been joyfully looking forward to his scheduled outing. He was not about to allow some bad weather to interfere with several hours of outside inter-action, and so off he went.

Meanwhile several volunteers sat on the couch holding babies. I could read in every one of their faces that they were just as concerned as I was. My friend Doneece actually asked if I thought we should move the pack and plays away from the window. None of us had ever experienced such odd weather.

Still worried, but multitasking as always, I decided to squeeze in a shower while volunteers lingered to wait out the storm. I took just a few minutes, enjoying the soothing spray of the water, but as I stepped out and began to dry my hair, I felt a pressing need to turn off the dryer and pray. At that time I had never really experienced what some call that "still small voice." It felt a bit dramatic—even for me, and wanting to get back to the babies, I tried to ignore the feeling and continued to dry my hair.

It didn't work. It was as if God was saying, "Are you listening to me?" I felt an indescribable urge to stop immediately and pray. Turn-ing to the twins who were playing just outside the bathroom door, I called to them, saying, "Girls, come! We need to ask Jesus to protect Daddy!" They scampered over and together we whispered a short but sincere prayer.

Not two minutes later, the phone rang. It was Jon. He breathlessly recounted to me how he had just driven through a tornado! He saw fields of corn to his left where the stalks stood steadfast and upright, while on the opposite side of the same road, they looked as if they had just been cut down by a giant sickle! An entire neighborhood in the small town of Palmyra had suffered severe damage as the funnel touched down.

I learned that day to heed that still small voice. Sometimes there is so much white noise humming in my ears that I can't hear what God is trying to tell me. I need to listen intently, and then most importantly, obey.

All in all, our first few weeks out of the hospital went fairly smoothly. It was like learning a complicated dance routine, and after many hours of practice, we slowly managed to nail down the first few steps. I knew there would be many tough days ahead. What I didn't realize was that going home would stir up a whole new set of feelings for me. In the condo, my natural tendency to sort of claim my space had not really kicked in; we were on neutral territory, and so streams of people coming in and out at all hours of the day and night, although anything but normal, was not nearly as unsettling as it would soon become when all of those people, some of them complete strangers, were standing in *my* house, in *my* family room, holding *my* babies.

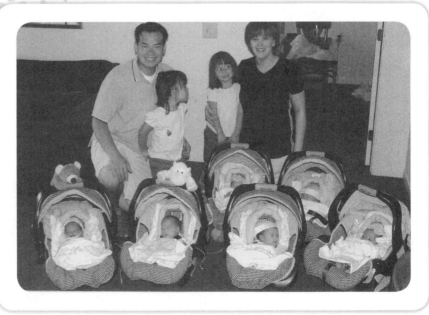

Going home as a family of ten—finally!

10 There's No Place Like Home

Even the sparrow has found a home,
    and the swallow a nest for herself,
    where she may lay her young.

Psalm 84:3

On the morning of July 18, I looked around the condo. It had served us well as our home away from home, and I wanted to imprint that crazy season of our lives in my memory. Long gone was the clean, clutter-free, hotel-like feel that greeted us five weeks previously. In its place were pack and plays, stacks of diapers and wipes, baby clothes, bottles, and blankets. It looked—and smelled—like six babies lived there. The many diaper changes tainted the air, but when I stood still for just a minute, I could also pick up the faint sweet scent of bath time mixed with the natural intoxicating perfume that newborns exude.

We had certainly taken over the rooms of the condo, leaving our impression everywhere I looked, but it was now time to move on. We were scheduled to return home the very next day. The task of packing up almost six months of accumulated belongings was daunting. I would pack some items, feed a baby, pump some milk, make some bottles, pack a box, feed the girls, change a baby, pump some milk, feed a baby, pack a box. Needless to say, even with volunteers helping with the babies and Jon jumping in to pack the big things, I had to once again dig deep to find the energy and drive just to keep going.

Besides the physical energy needed to get all ten of us packed, we had mental anxiety that occasionally threatened to cross the borderline into unrestrained panic. We had no form of transportation to take our babies home. I pictured us having to make two or more trips in our minivan. How else would all of the car seats and all of the stuff fit? Fortunately Jon's mom was thinking clearly and had called the producers of the home show that was busy finishing up the renovations on our house. The plan was that they would send a stretch limousine to carry our family home and then have the cameras rolling as we saw the big reveal for the first time. We were grateful.

But there was another problem: Besides the ten of us, there would also need to be one volunteer for each baby to ensure that feedings were not overlooked, diaper changes took place, monitors were carefully heeded, and basically no one or no thing fell through the cracks. I also wanted an additional volunteer to be solely responsible for Mady and Cara. It was bound to be an emotional and hectic day, and it was not smart or fair to expect them to just tag along. All of that brought our grand total to seventeen people.

The whole thing was beginning to look more and more like a three-ring circus. I remember as a kid watching the tightrope walker as the main event in the center ring of "The Greatest Show on Earth." It gave me great comfort then to see the nearly invisible net stretched out beneath him to catch him gently should he fall. As an adult, knowing that all eyes were on me that day, wanting directions, asking questions, even filming my response, I wanted to scream, "Lord, where's the net? Please be my net!"

Finally a plan was devised that covered all our bases. Jon and I held a small meeting in the living room of our condo to discuss our strategy with our main group of seven volunteers who would accompany us home that day. The plan was that all of our belongings would be packed in the limousine while all babies and volunteers would ride in another fifteen passenger van belonging to a friend, Jeff Brown, the father of quintuplets who lived in the area. He had graciously come to our rescue. Since it promised to be a long day and some volunteers would need to return to their own families, we had a group of backup volunteers lined up in four other vehicles to join our caravan. On paper it might seem like overkill, but stand in the midst of six hungry infants in the middle of a steamy July day with six months' worth of suitcases to unpack and camera crews coaxing a smile, and I think you would agree—backups were very necessary. God had graciously provided my net.

July 19 dawned, and the humidity clung to us like a wet blanket as everybody and everything was finally loaded up and ready to go. I decided I would sit in the very back seat of the van to be sure I could see each baby facing me should any of them need anything. I let my head rest on the seatback as I gave myself a pep talk for the hundredth time that day. Closing my eyes for just a minute, I could still see the index cards that my mother had hung all over my hospital room to comfort and encourage me. My favorite one had been from Matthew 11:28, which says, "Come to me, all you who are weary and burdened, and I will give you rest." I didn't think there could possibly be a more fitting verse for my condition at the time. What I didn't realize then was that that verse would resonate with meaning for me far beyond the actual physical delivery. Yes, I could finally see my feet again, but my head and my heart felt heavier than ever, weighed down by the awesome responsibilities and expectations that never subsided.

The drive went smoothly until I had to lift Collin out of his car seat just a few minutes from our driveway. His waning color was scaring me, and I knew he needed to be roused by touch and movement. As I jostled him awake, we turned onto our normally quiet suburban street, and I could hardly believe my eyes. It looked like a summer block party. Neighbors had gathered in the street and were excitedly snapping pictures and clapping as we pulled up to the house. The television camera crew had set up camp on the front lawn and was hurriedly getting into position. I just thought to myself, "Well, here we go."

●

Not five minutes after we stepped out of the vans, we had controversy. The television crew, wanting to capture my first reaction to the renovations, didn't want to bring the babies into the house until after they had the chance to film just Jon and me walking in. Well, that was a problem. Like any new mom, I couldn't wait to carry each baby into our home, welcoming each one and cherishing the memory. Besides that, it was a sweltering summer day and I didn't feel comfortable knowing my newborns would be sitting out in the van, even though it was air-conditioned. After firmly stating that the babies would indeed be going into the house, I did compromise by agreeing to the crew's request that the volunteers be the ones to walk the babies up to their room. It made me sad to step aside like a bystander as I watched the parade of car seats file by me on the way to a room that I couldn't even picture.

The volunteers were then told that they should come right back out so filming could begin. I shook my head thinking I had just misunderstood. Could I really be expected to allow my six premature infants, two still wearing monitors, to be alone in a room with no supervision for who knows how long? Again, we had a problem. Jon and I stood firm. The volunteers stayed or all cameras left. Period. Realizing we were not going to budge, the producer reluctantly nodded agreement but insisted that the door to the upstairs bedroom remain closed so no part of the makeover was revealed too early.

As I stood on the front steps of my home waiting for the signal to open the door, I wrestled with crashing waves of emotion as I prepared to step across the threshold of the home I hadn't seen in months. When I had left for the hospital, I had no idea what our lives would look like after the babies were born. Six months later, as I walked into our new living room, it hit me — I still had no idea what our lives looked like. Everything was different, even our home.

As I am sure those who were present can attest, I didn't know how to react. I had been told they were looking for that "million dollar reaction." I think I gave something that was a bit closer to a deer caught in the headlights. And then my eyes settled on one thing in the room: Hanging on the wall directly facing me was a photograph taken just after the babies were born by a local artist and owner of Willow Street Pictures.

I couldn't tear my eyes away from that black and white picture. It somehow captured the love and joy Jon and I felt as we sat looking, enamored by the abundance of our eight amazing blessings. I felt a hot tear roll down my cheek as I realized Collin's tiny little fingers of his left hand were splayed against his daddy's black shirt in the well-known position of "I love you" in sign language.

Realizing the crew was still holding their breath for my reaction, I was able to finally take in the rest of the room. The living room had

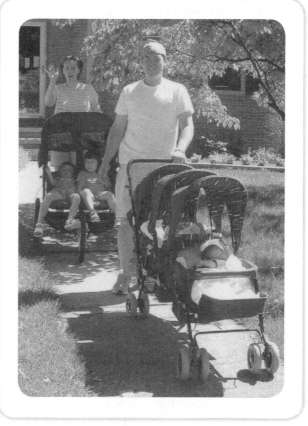

Our first family walk
(two babies in each seat of one triple stroller).

been nicely redecorated and painted, giving it a fresh, new modern feel. The kitchen also had seen major changes with much needed counter and storage space added. About six steps down on the lower level of our house, the two car garage had been converted to a master bedroom for Jon and me. I was thrilled to have a real bedroom set! It had been something I always wanted, but it never seemed to make it to the top of our list.

Next came the real surprise. We had not previously discussed any changes to Mady and Cara's bedroom or the babies' nursery, so I was mildly concerned when I was led up to the second floor. We stood first

There's No Place Like Home •

at the babies' closed door to the left of the stairs. I was envisioning a peaceful, restful color on the walls with the cribs lined up neatly and all their little clothes folded cleanly and put away. The door opened and I was taken aback. The room had been painted in what I considered to be garish primary colors and almost frighteningly large illustrations of nursery rhyme figures. The cribs were lined up in rows with alternating changing tables between each of them, allowing just a narrow strip of walking space between each row. The room was so loud and overcrowded; it perfectly exemplified the overwhelming, screaming insanity of our situation.

I couldn't help it: I cried. I don't think hysterically sobbing fell under the description of "million dollar reaction." I just couldn't imagine my tiny five-pound babies coming from the pristine and deliberately calm environment of the NICU to the stuffy, fussy, overstimulating room that I was standing in.

Taking a deep breath, I tried to regain my composure in hopes of smoothing some very ruffled feathers. However, as I next walked into Mady and Cara's room, I just lost it. I felt the blood drain from my face as I stood in a room that once had been covered in a sweet pastel print — something I thought to be very fitting for three-year-old twin girls. The room had been painted in wide purple stripes with huge orange daisies dancing along the walls. Again, what struck a nerve was that when I had left my house, my girls were just coming out of toddlerhood. Suddenly, I felt like I was entering a room more fitting for girls approaching their teen years. Could I really have missed that much?

The bottom line was that I had reached my saturation limit for change. I was unable to take in yet another surprise. Not being one to hide my feelings well, my face said it all, and I'm afraid I came across as an ungrateful brat. It wasn't so much that I was disagreeing about color choices; I was simply reeling from constant adjustments. I just wanted to scream "Stop!" It was never my intention to end the day on such a sour note. I realize that many, many people worked long hours to do something that they felt would make my transition easier. In fact, most of the changes did make it possible for us to survive the next year in that small house on a tree-lined street in Wyomissing, and for that I am eternally grateful.

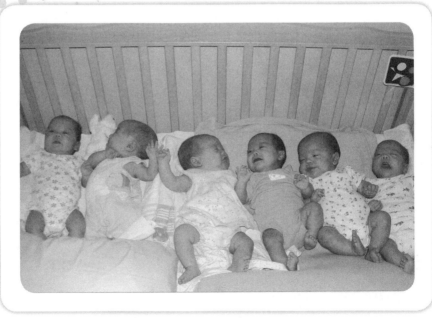

Baby lineup at three months. Left to right:
Leah, Aaden, Alexis, Hannah, Collin, and Joel.

11 Who Are All These People?

And my God will meet all your needs according to
his glorious riches in Christ Jesus.

Philippians 4:19

Our first day in our home as a family had not exactly gone as I
had hoped. After my meltdown, the camera crew left in a hurry,
leaving food, water bottles, and coffee cups behind in their wake. There
were no heartfelt good-byes, and tension was high between Jon, his
mother, and me.

I knew I had not been the perfect picture of graciousness, and yet
I could not muster anything but disgust as I watched a few of the
volunteers silently wiping the thick layer of dust off the silverware and
dishes in the kitchen so we could have some dinner. I had left my house
immaculately clean, and I was disappointed to not find it just as clean
when I returned.

Little things that maybe shouldn't have made me crumble—such
as the heaping load of disheveled items that tumbled out of the babies'
closet the first time I opened the doors—became monumental in the
midst of so much stress.

By four o'clock in the afternoon new volunteers had begun to filter in.
Most of them were people who had responded to a request for help in our
church bulletin or who had somehow learned of our plight through the
media or a friend. By then the women who had been there all day were still
running the dishwasher in the kitchen and doing their best to help keep
the babies on schedule and Cara and Mady to a respectable volume.

I noticed an undertow of territorial behavior as the experienced volunteers were forced to hand the baton to new people whom they had never met. That was not as easy as it sounds. I had a set routine that I was absolutely adamant about instituting from the beginning. It started at the front door. Every volunteer or visitor, whether there for two minutes or two hours, whether lifetime friend or complete stranger, would first remove her shoes and leave them by the door. Second, she would be expected to head upstairs to the small pink bathroom down the hall from the nursery and thoroughly scrub her hands with soap from the NICU. The third stop was back down to the closet by the front door where she would find a variety of clean hospital scrubs from which to choose to wear over her top. I preferred long hair to be tied back and no heavy perfume to be worn. I know I sound like a holy terror at war against germs. I was called names and criticized to no end for being an over-the-top, neurotic drill sergeant, but I do not apologize for one minute. I was on a single-minded mission to protect my fragile babies from the onslaught of potential health threats that were carried in by sometimes twenty to twenty-five people every single day.

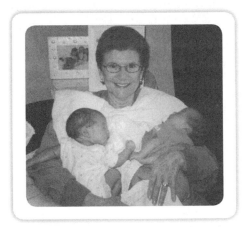

Nanny Joan with Hannah and Leah.

We set up baby base camp in the family room, which was in the lower level of the house. A large black sectional stretched around the room in front of an entertainment center. We moved one of the changing tables down from the nursery, along with one crib, to the far corner of the family room, next to the door leading outside. My goal was to provide a workable space for the night nurses so they would not have to tromp up and down the uncarpeted stairs all night long to retrieve and deposit babies into cribs. It was medically unsafe for them to sleep unattended; besides, all six babies were quite content, and adorable I might add, to snuggle up all in a row in just one crib.

About four days after we got home, Joan, a woman who had been present at Jon's birth and had babysat him when he was young, showed up at our door. I knew instantly by looking at her strong yet smiley and capable exterior that her heartbeat was to be a helper. She took one look at "Little Lovely Leah," as she was later named by "Nanny Joan," and that was it.

Joan quickly became a fixture at feeding times. She would quietly step through the front door, slip off her shoes, and peek her head down the stairs to the family room. "Any babies for me?" she'd call. She readily volunteered to be the brave one to coax our tiny Leah through four labor-intensive ounces at each feeding. The real problem wasn't that Leah wouldn't eat; it was that Joan usually ending up wearing those four ounces all over her green scrub jacket that she claimed as her own from the closet. Leah had severe issues with acid reflux and therefore had projectile vomiting after most feedings. It didn't even faze Joan as she had had a daughter with the same problems. She unceremoniously prepared what would become known as "Joan's corner" which was a section of the couch that she had draped with sheets to protect the cushions as much as possible from the inevitable onslaught. In front of her was always a shallow yellow bowl from the hospital that sat on a small square wooden pedestal table. It was within arm's reach for Joan to grasp when she knew Leah would need it.

Joan's talents didn't stop at baby soothing and vomit cleaning. She also appointed herself "Queen of Consignment." With bags and bags of clothing items being dropped off by anyone who had ever had a child it seemed, it soon became a necessity to carefully edit or be buried alive in onesies and sleepers. Joan sat and went through each bag, carefully choosing the items that were in the best condition and were the correct sizes. She then consolidated any items that were not needed and packed them up to take to a local kids' consignment store. She convinced me that the extra money was necessary with Jon still out of work, and people who wanted to help would be happy that the clothing, even though not worn by the babies, had definitely aided us in some way.

Another volunteer, Beth, arrived at my door one afternoon for the four o'clock feeding. She, like so many other complete strangers, was quickly taken through the basic routine. She hesitated for just a second, however, to slip a white envelope onto the kitchen counter before going down to the family room. As I didn't have the time or the desire to chat and make friends with her, or anyone frankly, I simply tucked the envelope away in my "someday when I have time" pile that was growing by the phone. Meanwhile, weeks passed and Beth arrived regularly to feed a baby, and occasionally, especially at nighttime feedings, we would actually have the time to talk and get to know each other. Finally one day, I read what was in the envelope. Opening it, I found a handwritten letter, telling me who my new friend was — a devoted wife, mother, and Christian. More important, it was refreshing to hear that she understood how strange and uncomfortable it must feel to hand my babies over to pretty much anyone who walked through the front door. Beth soon became my mentor, my sounding board, and my coach as I walked this seemingly hopeless and lonely road.

Our financial situation was beginning to look bleak. Jon continually searched for job opportunities but was told he was either overqualified or underqualified. He was exhausted and frustrated, but I think the hardest part was being constantly surrounded with a roomful of female volunteers who would unknowingly take a stab at his male ego every time they asked the inevitable question of the day, "So Jon, did you find a job yet?" I'd cringe every time because I knew he felt like a failure who could not provide for his family.

One night, he just broke down in tears as he put on his coat to go run some errands. As the front door closed, I prayed as I sat on the couch feeding a baby, that he would come home to us and not just keep driving away as far as he could go. I didn't need to worry. He came back that night, eyes red from lack of sleep and a good cry, and he jumped right back in, picking up a swaddled baby and tenderly tucking him in for the night. He had decided he would take the only opportunity he had at that moment to make some money; he would apply to be an aide in the local school district.

Joan, who worked at the high school, knew they needed substitutes on a fairly regular basis. The burning question though was if it was really worth the measly fifty dollars a day that Jon would earn in exchange for the stability and extra set of capable hands he offered at home. It was certainly a toss-up, but he did go when they called because, at that point, it wasn't only about the money. It was a small escape into reality with real people with whom to interact. As an extrovert, that was important for Jon. It kept him from falling into depression.

Meanwhile, I had my own hurdles to clear. My severely atrophied muscles still made it difficult to carry out even the most mundane of daily tasks. Regardless, with six feedings a day, I became like a mad chemist in the kitchen, mixing thirty-six bottles each and every morning. I would stumble out to the stovetop, still half asleep, and fill two huge Pyrex measuring cups with fresh water to be boiled. After it cooled I would get out my plastic Rubbermaid half gallon shaker and shake, shake, shake till my arms were tired. I had to keep in mind that I had Aaden, Collin, and Hannah who were on soy-based Isomil, thickened with just a bit of rice cereal; Alexis and Joel who had the same formula unthickened; and Leah on Alimentum, a milk-based formula that was easier to digest. I came up with a color-coded system to help me remember whose bottle was whose. Hannah was pink; Leah, green; Aaden, yellow; Collin, blue; Joel, red; and Alexis, purple. I would add all of my pumped breast milk from the day (splitting it six ways again) and their Poly-Vi-Sol infant vitamin to their 8:00 p.m. bottle, making it easier to also add some rice since breast milk is so much thinner than formula.

Who Are All These People? •

I stuck a toothpick in the nipple of each nighttime bottle to allow the thickened formula to pass through easier.

I cleared one entire shelf of our refrigerator. Taped under each neatly lined up row of plastic bottles was a small yellow sticky note with the time of each feeding and an arrow, preventing random bottles from being grabbed and consequently wreaking havoc on my system.

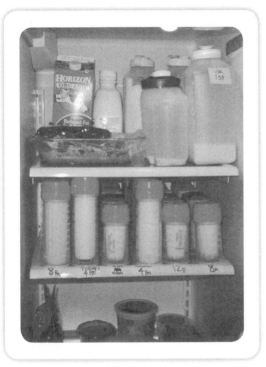

Bottle shelf in the refrigerator.

One thing I learned that I strongly suggest to mothers of multiples is to choose bottles with disposable liners. It may cost a bit more but it will save you many late night appointments with the bottle brush. Sometimes time is more valuable than actual money.

Several weeks after being home, observant volunteers offered to take over my tedious bottle-making task. While it was certainly tempting, I actually enjoyed my kitchen duties for the most part. Since cooking for my family is a passion and something that gives me great pleasure, I considered those bottles to be akin to a well-made dinner. It would make me proud to walk down to the family room carrying another yellow hospital bowl — they were really handy — filled with freshly warmed bottles. Someone once quipped, "Hey kids, hang on now. Here comes the Dairy Queen!" It made me happy to think that I really put thought and effort into each baby's dietary requirements and went the extra mile to ensure they were satisfied each day.

Bottle confusion was really the least of my worries however. With money and nerves stretched taut, I felt more and more cornered and vulnerable. My whole existence had become a double-edged sword. On the one hand, I wanted so badly to do it myself. On the other hand, I knew that my pride had to be shelved because I was completely at the mercy of the kindness of so many people in order to survive. I found myself praying in a new and different way. I had always been taught reverence for God, but now it had matured into a deep and personal relationship. I felt like I had a heavenly Father who would meet all my needs and listen to every cry from my heart. I could almost feel the Lord carrying me through the rough spots much like in the popular poem, "Footprints in the Sand."

At one point, with the entire country reeling from the drastic increase in the price of oil, our monthly expenses to heat our small home actually tripled. We were forced to keep the temperature in our home extremely low. So low, in fact, we put our newborns to bed with onesies, heavy pajamas, socks, fleece slippers, vests, and even hats. Again, the only thing I could do was pray.

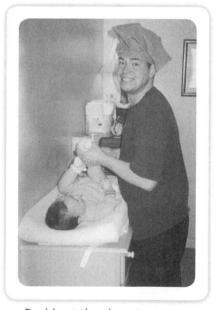

Daddy at the changing station with Alexis's pants on his head for safekeeping.

Some of those prayers were answered in the form of generous donations that continued to pour in. Besides the many items like six cribs, two triple-wide strollers, and six Graco car seats, just to name a few, there were others—like five thousand dollars in gift cards and a year's supply of diapers donated by Giant grocery stores. Our local store even went so far as to hang a cute sign with a picture of a stork on one of the closest parking places in their lot. It said "Reserved for the Gosselin Gosslings." Also, Lucky Leaf and

Musselman's Corporation donated a lifetime supply of applesauce and apple juice.

Smaller companies got in on the action also. In September, I received a phone call from Bob, my Allstate insurance agent, himself a father of six children. He wondered if we could set up a meeting because he had something he wanted to present to us. It turned out to be a check for fifteen hundred dollars, six soft white blankets, a monetary donation in our name to the Ronald McDonald House, and one promise. The promise was to try his best to have one year of our car insurance wiped clean from our growing slate of bills. It took several months, but the bills did indeed stop coming.

Every time I felt like I was going to crack from the pressure of mounting bills, it seemed as though God would strategically place someone in my path to remind me He was there. There was a business in Harrisburg, Pennsylvania, called C.J. Pony Parts, a distributor of Ford Mustang parts. Jon and I used to laugh out loud and make a funny comment like, "Who would buy pony parts?" every time we passed that store. We were surprised later that winter with a Christmas card from that very place, which contained a five-hundred-dollar gift certificate to Target and a five-hundred-dollar gift certificate to Giant.

There were generous people like the family from my sister Kendra's church, people whom I had never met, who sent us a check for six thousand dollars. I dropped to my knees sobbing when I opened it, as that check paid our mortgage until Jon was able to finally get a job.

A group of women at the place where one of my cousins worked decided to host a baby shower on my behalf. One volunteer named Rita would faithfully leave a fifty-dollar bill on the open schedule book I left on the kitchen counter for volunteers to sign up in. She knew our needs were great, she said, and just wanted to help. Just like the person who one Sunday morning left a white envelope on the buffet in my living room. I opened it, and again sobbed as five hundred dollars slipped out.

I never learned who left that money, although I questioned almost everyone who came in for the next week. It seemed no one knew. But I knew: it was yet another angel sent by God to show His love. I knew I did not deserve His grace or His mercy, but He unconditionally doled it out anyway. I tucked those moments away,

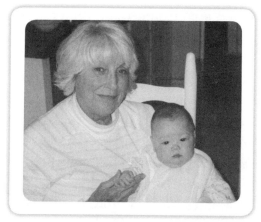

Nanna Janet and Alexis

at first unable to scrutinize God's motives. As I had more time to digest it all, I realized that God was showing me a picture of what He wanted me to become. Because I was raised in an atmosphere of financial stress, my biggest fear was that I would never have enough. God was slowly erasing those fears and taking me full circle to realize that not only did I not need as much as I once thought I did to exist, but that He would in fact never be late in meeting my needs. If I just trusted Him, He would give me more fulfillment than I ever thought possible. Wow.

With that thought in mind, I'd like to take this opportunity to personally thank each and every one of you, and you know who you are, for every single gift ever offered to my family. Whether it was a cooked meal, precious clothes, a smile for Mady and Cara, money in any amount, work on our house, supplies for the babies, or that most precious of commodities these days—your time—Jon and I thank you from the bottom of our hearts. Many notes of gratitude never made it from my list to the mailbox; it was not for lack of appreciation but merely lack of time. May you all be blessed a hundredfold for your generosity.

In September, Cara and Mady were absolutely thrilled to attend preschool. Somehow in a lucid moment way back in March, I realized they would need the interaction and escape by the time fall approached. I made a phone call to the director of Lakeside Early Learning Center and was told there were just two spots open. Hesitating for just a moment, not exactly certain how in the world we were going to afford preschool times two, I took a leap of faith and said, "We'll take them!" Explaining my situation to the director, we decided that cutting the girls' attendance from three days a week down to two days would alleviate a bit of the financial strain while still allowing the girls to reap the many benefits of preschool.

Months later as I drove the girls to school one day, I could see the decision to commit one hundred and fifty dollars a month of our miniscule budget was well worth it. The girls had been literally bouncing around the condo and then the house for months on end. We were all a little stir-crazy, and getting them out to be challenged and stimulated was good for everyone.

I decided that I wanted to be the one to take them to school twice a week in the morning. I felt like I at least had to do that one "normal mommy" thing for them, and just as importantly, it gave the three of us a few minutes alone together. It took a huge amount of planning as I had to be sure to have all the bottles ready and waiting when the volunteers showed up to help Jon with the morning feeding.

The girls loved their preschool experience, although it made me acutely aware of how different our lives were compared to other families. "You forgot to send a snack again, like all the other mommies did," Mady dramatically reminded me one day. I knew there were many ways I was not like "all the other mommies," and school snacks would not be the only thing that didn't make my list some days. I had to deal with these minor disappointments as well as to teach Mady and Cara to do the same.

I was surprised at how awkward I felt as I stood in the hallway with all the other moms. I would longingly watch a young mom lugging in a car seat with a sleepy infant nestled in for a nap or another mom who chatted with her toddler who wound around her legs clutching a favorite blanket and sucking her thumb. I wondered if I would ever have the chance, the time, to do even those most common everyday mommy things.

I couldn't even talk about my babies as other moms told funny stories or shared mothering tips. Whenever I did mention that no, Mady and Cara, were not my only children, that I, in fact, had six infants waiting at home, dead silence followed. All eyes turned to me and the floodgates were opened. I was immediately pelted with question after question, with expressions of disbelief and shock. I felt like the freak show at the county fair. Sometimes, though, it was a relief to sort of let the cat out of the bag and actually admit that my home was filled to the brim with living, breathing miracles.

In October, as the leaves started turning colors, the babies also were changing. They no longer needed to be tightly swaddled as they once loved to be. Even though they were six months old, they were more like three-month-olds, and the world was just beginning to look more interesting to them. Cara and Mady were capable little helpers, distinguishing each baby's cry from another and proudly reciting each name in a quick review for volunteers whenever asked.

While the girls loved to move from volunteer to volunteer, telling stories, singing songs, and generally enjoying the attention, I often felt sorry for them. Some days they would just hit a wall. They were used to being the stars of the show, the loves of our lives, and the princesses in every respect. How could they not feel like extras on an overcrowded set being constantly pushed aside for their new younger co-stars? Mady would get angry and act out, scowling and stamping her little foot with indigence, while Cara had a sadness in her eyes when she inevitably had to wait her turn for something.

In a determined attempt to carve out an afternoon for Mady and Cara to stand proudly in the undivided spotlight, I decided to throw a fourth birthday party for them in the backyard. Birthday parties were a huge tradition in our house. They were into Strawberry Shortcake at the time, and I was thrilled to have a special cake made that looked just like her straw hat. There were balloons, games, and streamers, but more important, there was the noticeable absence of bottles, diapers, and crying. I purposely arranged for Jon to drop off all the babies at Joan and Terry's house with several volunteers for the afternoon. Packing them all up, getting the food prepared, and trying to add a few festive touches basically took every bit as much planning and effort as the previous year's trip to Disney World, which already seemed like a lifetime ago. It was the time in our lives when even taking a shower was a huge accomplishment; there simply weren't enough hours in a day to fit everything in. I know some people thought it was ludicrous to squeeze a party into our lives at that time, but the smiles on Mady's and Cara's faces that afternoon told me it had been a wise investment. For just a few hours, they shed their big-sister status and ran around in the grass with silly four-year-old abandon.

●

As the babies' world was expanding, ours seemed to be getting smaller and smaller. Jon and I felt isolated even though we were exposed and on public display. It was humiliating to have very personal discussions, especially concerning our money situation, Jon's lack of employment, discipline of the girls, or even personal trials and feelings, in front of whoever happened to be helping with the babies at any given moment. Many times I would explode at Jon, making him the dartboard for all my anger, fear, and frustration. Our five years of marriage felt like a thin crust of ice on a frozen pond. Even minor disagreements seemed to put major cracks in the ice, and I was afraid one of us was just going to fall through one day and drown.

Already feeling defeated and overwhelmed, I answered a phone call one morning from an old friend from nursing school. She called to break the news to me that Melissa, my best friend and roommate in nursing school, had been killed that afternoon in a car accident. My mind screamed and spun as I strained to hear the words "not wearing her seatbelt," and "her nineteen-month-old was found strapped in his car seat unharmed." I completely crumbled. Melissa was a sweet, sensitive friend and mother, and I couldn't digest the cruel reality of her untimely death. I had been lamenting my truly blessed situation when

her dear family was living the ultimate nightmare. I stumbled down the stairs blinded by tears, to find Jon — my husband, my voice of comfort, my faithful tower of strength. We might have sometimes fought like two old cranky rivals, but when all else was peeled away, we always found each other to be standing side by side, devoted and committed.

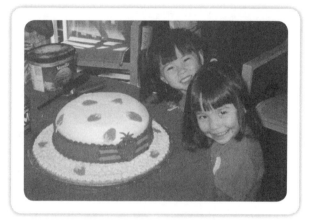

Cara and Mady with their fourth birthday hat cake.

On the day of Melissa's funeral, Jon and I left all eight kids in the care of volunteers. I had the kitchen and family room littered with Post-it reminders about everything from hand washing to which bottles to give first during bedtime routines. With red eyes and heavy hearts, we closed our front door on the deafening chorus of hungry, crying babies. Our first "date night" was not anything close to what I had envisioned. I felt like I could barely walk from the weight of sorrow and grief mixed with my own murky world of complex emotions.

Melissa's death was like someone throwing a bucket of cold water on the first few sparks of my reinvented life that I had been desperately trying to fan into flame. Sadness smothered me, clouding my vision and dampening my outlook. As so often happens, sadness, mixed with the turmoil of everyday life, spilled over into, "Why me?" Before I knew it, I was wallowing neck deep in self-pity. I felt guilty even having those feelings because I realized it was all relative. How could I possibly compare my daily trials to the gaping hole in the heart of Melissa's family? Isn't this what I had always wanted—to be a stay-at-home mom, to have my three kids, dishes, laundry, and noise? So what if I might've gotten a whole lot more than I bargained for? I was supposedly living my dream, right?

Still, I fought off depression as I lay in bed one morning, already hearing volunteers in the family room but wanting to just bury my head and never get up. I could hear snippets of their conversation, everyday happy things like the new restaurant they visited, a niece's much anticipated wedding, "Oh, I must get a pedicure!" and oohs and ahhs over a stylish new haircut.

I wondered to myself, "Can't anyone see that I am bleeding over here?" To me it felt like I was a gunshot victim lying in a pool of blood on the floor of the emergency room while everyone rushed out to clip a hangnail. I became very resentful as I listened to the pointless chatter; at the time it all seemed so shallow. I know, I know. You're asking if I really thought the entire world would stop because I had six babies and two preschoolers. The answer is no. What I did think was that *my* world had stopped. I know today that that was not the case at all. Actually, my life was really just beginning. But at the time, I felt that though we had cribs, car seats, pretty new paint, dressers, food, financial support from so many—not to mention eight very healthy, happy children—we would never be "normal" again.

My sharp and cynical attitude was not winning me any friends in the circle of volunteers. A few were perceptive enough to add up the hormonal plunge, the lack of sleep, the all-consuming and never-ending responsibility, the loss of my dear friend, and the worry over the mounting pile of unpaid bills to explain my moodiness; but most would just eye me warily as they slunk past my post at the kitchen counter on their way down to the family room. As I prepared bottles and a meal for Mady and Cara, I would get tears in my eyes. I had never before realized it was possible to feel so alone in the midst of so many people.

I began to feel like an outsider in my own home as small social cliques were formed among some of the volunteers. I noticed that several people actually hung around well after the baby they had been feeding was sleeping and could be tucked into bed. They'd discuss their various viewpoints on everything from a great sale at Boscov's to who had cramps that week to how to get that darn husband of theirs to pick up his dirty laundry. I would often sit with a glazed look in my eyes trying to remember when I actually thought any of those topics worthy of that much discussion. I was usually too tired to comment.

I loved the time of the night when I would actually sit and snuggle one of my babies instead of looking at the clock and needing to move onto the next chore. It was often the one and only time throughout the day when I could actually observe and appreciate the little things about my babies. It didn't surprise me one bit that Collin, by far the biggest, was all about his food, always the first one to be finished, down to the last drop. Meanwhile, Aaden fussed and fidgeted, sometimes also down to the last drop. Alexis, happy with the first few ounces, found it plain troublesome to bother with the last few ounces at all, and would promptly fall asleep.

Usually it became "Nanna" Janet's job to keep our little Alexis on task. Janet brought much laughter and silly antics to the comparatively sedate crowd. Jon and I agree that Janet's crazy form of boundless joy had to have rubbed off on Alexis during all those hours spent bonding over bottles. Alexis is now a mini-Janet in many ways—loud, giggly, loving, and the life of any party.

As the last of the babies finished his or her evening bottle, Jon would silently lift each warm, sleepy little bundle out of the arms of the volunteer, then walk over to me, and put a soft damp baby cheek up to my face for a good-night kiss. It was those moments when I would see the angelic expression of a fed, freshly diapered, content baby that kept me sane.

At that time, we had three pack and plays consuming every available space in our small bedroom; two were wedged next to the dresser under the window and one was on the other side of the room right by the door. It was important to me to have the babies close by so I could hear their soft breathing as I fell into bed, usually by 10:30 each night. Later in the darkness, as they woke up for their midnight feeding, I'd hear one of the nurses tiptoe in and lift a crying baby out of his crib. The room would gradually grow quieter as one by one, all six were fed and then put back to sleep out in the family room. With the final rotation of the day completed, I would finally fall into a deep sleep for the last few remaining hours of the night.

Jon, on the other hand, wary of people strolling around the house and taking care of our babies, was still in the habit of staying awake and helping the nurses to make sure each baby's needs were met. I thought sometimes he had become so accustomed to carrying the weight of the world on his shoulders that he almost couldn't turn himself off. As the months of no paychecks wore on, I grew more and more worried about him. People commented on how exhausted he looked; his eyes were red-rimmed, his hair uncharacteristically messy, his face unshaven, and his sweatpants a uniform.

That was not the Jon I knew. Normally he was neurotic about his clothes being pressed, face clean-shaven, and being well groomed. Now at times he just stared blankly as he sat holding two restless babies or he slumped at the computer, filling out countless job applications. I needed him, and watching him run himself into the ground was like watching a speeding racecar about to spin out of control. The worst part was that we were in this figurative car together; if he crashed and burned, so did the rest of us. I knew that no one felt that pressure more acutely than Jon. I loved him for each minute that he managed to hold it together for the sake of our family.

●

In November, another crazy curveball was thrown our way. Jon's father had been suffering with heart issues for quite some time by then. He was diabetic and his health had deteriorated significantly since the birth of the babies. While he still managed to work at his pediatric dentistry office, frequent hospital visits became the norm.

When we were notified that he was admitted to the hospital yet again, I think we were in denial about the fact that his health had gone from bad to worse. Jon's dad, Poppy, as the girls knew him, was an integral part of our everyday life. He would stop in daily for a visit, always unveiling a little surprise while Mady and Cara danced around him with their little hands held out in anticipation. It would usually be as simple as a few coins from his pocket for their piggy banks, but it was delivered with such genuine kindness and affection that it always made the girls beam with love for their Poppy. One look at the smile on Poppy's face and even complete strangers could see that the feeling was mutual. His biggest role in life was being a good grandfather.

When the babies were born, he proudly displayed pictures and newspaper clippings in his office for all to see. He had renewed vigor, and I'd like to believe that in a time of his life when each breath became a hard-won battle, our tiny miracles winning their own battles gave him strength. Many times he'd just smile tenderly as he looked around at our lively crew. The unquenchable love and pride in his eyes when he was with our children was a true blessing to us, and we drew strength knowing that he was always there to offer whatever he could to help us.

When Poppy was moved to the Intensive Care Unit, Jon and I got nervous. We had been lulled into a pattern of hospitalizations followed by a recovery period, and then back to work as usual. We began to realize though that eventually one of those times, it wasn't going to end on such a good note. That day before we could leave for the hospital, we called several volunteers who had become our core group, a group who worked well together as a team and could reliably handle just about anything. They came to sit with the kids, and after we explained the situation, they shooed us out the door to go share some much needed private conversation with Jon's dad.

Being Christians, we believe that by accepting Christ as our personal Savior we are assured of spending eternity with Him in heaven. We wanted and needed to know that Jon's dad felt that peace. The three of us talked openly and freely for quite some time that night, and by the end of the visit, I felt somewhat comforted that his heart, while in poor shape physically, was growing stronger and stronger spiritually. In spite of being diagnosed with congestive heart failure and pneumonia, Poppy once again rallied, was discharged from the hospital, and even returned to his dentistry practice on a part-time basis.

We, in the meantime, kept plugging along, each day praying for a break that would bring Jon a job. I would vacillate between complete trust that surely God had a plan, and raging, angry fear and despair. The coinciding ups and downs of Jon's dad's life and ours were a shared roller-coaster ride none of us wanted to be on.

On the day before Thanksgiving, right after the four o'clock feeding, I caught a glimpse of three people standing on my front doorstep as I passed by the front window. Curious, I went to the door and found three of Jon's dad's longtime colleagues about to ring the doorbell. They looked apologetic and explained that they hadn't wanted to disturb me but just wished to drop something off. I invited them in to see the babies who happened to be having one of those rare, quiet, and somewhat under control play times. With full bellies, they all happily sat either in Exersaucers or bouncy seats, or they rolled on blankets on the floor. I kind of giggled at the awestruck look on my visitors' faces as they stood on the stairs awkwardly leaning into the room. I could tell that it was a unique scene for them to take in; lots of flailing fingers and toes topped with slobbery baby noises and sprinkled with jingling dashes of colorful rattles and toys. I wanted to say, "Yeah, I know. Overwhelming."

It was a brief visit that once again ended in tears of thankfulness as I closed the front door. I couldn't believe it. With just a few weeks before Christmas, I held in my hand the most thoughtful two-part gift. First, a Celine Dion CD entitled *Miracles*; it had a touching photograph on the front cover of the tiniest baby held in a tender embrace. Second, a check for $1500. When I looked at the check with a questioning expression, Poppy's colleagues were quick to explain that they just wanted to do whatever they could to help. I was so touched.

I'll admit that not ten minutes before they arrived on my doorstep, I was not in the mood for Thanksgiving; my biggest focus was getting my third load of laundry folded and starting to prepare everyone for bed. Once again, while I was stuck in the moment, God, on the other hand, was seeing to the details of my future.

I don't think my visitors could've possibly understood what their gift meant to us; it meant we could pay our bills that month and perhaps even get a few small Christmas gifts for the girls. It also touched our hearts that people thought enough of Jon's dad that they would reach out to help his family; it was a tribute to Poppy's generous character.

On a frigid night in December, I set out for the local Target, armed with several gift cards we had received. I was thrilled at the adventure of being out of the house by myself. Although the babies had been home for months — they were seven months old at that time — I had not been out on my own even one time, and certainly not at night. I felt free and yet uneasy. Everything looked so different as I ventured toward the highway. Actually, everything *was* different. Not having read a newspaper or even listened to the local news in months, I was completely unaware that a major highway project, which included a new bypass, had been completed since the last time I drove that particular stretch of road. I was just five minutes from my home, yet I felt totally lost. I felt the darkness envelop me as my headlights anxiously searched the new green traffic signs looking for something familiar.

Suddenly I wished I had paid more attention to several conversations the volunteers had had concerning all of the recent changes. I just couldn't think. I felt a real kinship to how soldiers must feel as they are trained for battle by being deprived of sleep for long periods of time and then told to do a seemingly simple task. I was utterly lost less than two miles from home. Finally, I grudgingly called home and admitted to Jon, who pretty much thought I had permanently lost my mind, that I needed directions to a store I had been to maybe a hundred times before.

As Christmas approached, we held our breath as Jon awaited word about a job in Harrisburg, Pennsylvania, as an IT analyst for the state in Governor Rendell's office. After filling out possibly a hundred different applications, the job search looked very bleak — until the day when Jon received a phone call from Senator O'Pake. The senator had read about our situation and asked if there was any way at all he could be of help. When Jon told him about his frustrating job search and his latest application, the senator assured Jon that he would personally deliver the application to the capital to avoid any further delay in receiving a response.

Thanking him, Jon hung up the phone with a new dose of confidence. After hearing for months that he was either overqualified or underqualified, he knew that he was perfectly qualified for his latest quest. He even had his MCSE, Microsoft Certified Systems Engineer, credentials. Thankfully he had been persistent about taking the six-month course for two nights each week back when the girls were two years old. He hoped his increased depth of knowledge would give him an edge.

Jon and I enjoyed the most inspiring and encouraging experience each night as we walked around in the quiet aftermath of the final feeding. As I threw in a last load of laundry and moved on to kitchen duty, setting out formula, bibs, and lists for the next day, I would notice little things that had appeared in my kitchen throughout the busy day — things like a fresh box of Playtex bottle liners on the kitchen counter. A volunteer had placed them there realizing I was almost always running short. Sometimes there would be a plate of homemade cookies or other special treat carefully wrapped and waiting for me to discover.

Then I'd see Jon standing by the Christmas tree just shaking his head. Each day more and more small gifts appeared under that little tree without us ever knowing it, without a word ever being mentioned. I felt blessed and humbled that so many people were being used by God to make that Christmas one of the most memorable ever for my family. I knew He was seeing to our every need day by day. I still don't even know who left most of those gifts, but I thank you all and want you to know that my children will hear of the miracles of that Christmas each year as we think of the generosity of the many caring people who touched our lives.

It was a short time later when we received the best Christmas gift of all—Jon got the job at the state capital. He was offered the position and would begin his new career just after the start of the new year. Maybe, just maybe, we were on the way to settling down into some kind of routine. Maybe somehow we could reestablish our financial footing and regain at least some form of stability and security. Jon woke the next morning with a new confidence, a renewed hope and vision. It was like the whole house got a shot of adrenaline.

That shot of adrenaline didn't go far; late in December my father-in-law once again took a turn for the worse. He was admitted to Penn State Milton S. Hershey Medical Center and the news from the cardiologist was dismal: They had done everything they possibly could, and the end was sadly imminent.

Grieving over a loved one's suffering is difficult at best, but not understanding what is happening makes it even more stressful. I felt it my duty to Jon to help decipher all the medical jargon being thrown at us. It was difficult for him, and it made me feel that in a small way I could be of some help to Jon and his family, even though I obviously couldn't be at the hospital every day. I would put down a baby, bottle, diaper, dish, or basket of laundry long enough each morning to pay close attention to the latest information. Writing it all down on a tablet by the phone, I would then call Jon's two brothers, Tommy and Mark, and then Uncle Jerry and Aunt Diane to keep everyone up-to-date.

The downside of understanding certain medical red flags was that I carried the burden of preparing Jon for what lay ahead. I would take him aside and gently try to explain that he needed to be prepared; his father had begun to show signs of multi-organ failure. I didn't want Jon, distracted by the pressure of a brand new job on top of the never-ending demands at home, to be blindsided by his father's impending death. He really needed to take the signs at face value; it seemed that this time there would be no bouncing back as had been the case so many times in the past.

Just a few days before New Year's Day, as we sat feeding babies, Jon took a phone call from the doctor in Hershey. I watched my husband's shoulders slump as he was told that his father would be placed on life support before the end of the day. To this day I feel guilty for not just reaching over, taking the baby from his arms, and saying, "Just go!" I realized only later that I should've known that it would be Jon's last chance to ever visit with his dad without the image of the tangled web of equipment forever imprinting its ugly self on his memory.

My last conversation with Jon's dad had been over the phone on Christmas Day while the girls played quietly in their room with some of their newly opened gifts and the babies napped. A few moments of silence were very rare in our house, and I was so grateful to be able to speak to him without constant interruptions. His voice was gruff and rasping as he labored for breath. "I wish I was there with you," he said. Filled with emotion, I searched in vain for just the right words to say. How could I possibly express how thankful I was for the kind and generous father-in-law and grandfather he had been, his commitment to loving us and even providing for us during the most desperate of times during that year? He was always there. One time when he saw me crying over my stack of bills on the counter, he said, "Whatever it is Kate, just tell me. I'll help." That was his heart, and now that tender heart was failing him. It just didn't seem fair.

Jon spoke often with his dad and remembers his last real conversation with him while he was still able to communicate being in the parking lot of Sam's Club. Jon, having a full cart of household necessities, hurried to his car in the crowded lot packed with the onslaught of holiday grocery shoppers. Freezing in the biting wind as he struggled to unload the cart while fumbling with the phone, he just checked in with his dad but didn't talk long. Both father and son just assumed they would speak again later. Jon's father ended the conversation on that cold day in late December as he had so many times before—a simple "I love you."

We rejoiced at the promises of a new year as Jon started his new job at the state capital in Harrisburg. A heaviness hung in the air however, as Poppy lay in a hospital room on life support. Jon would stop at the hospital every day on his way home from work to spend time with his dad. My heart would ache for Jon as I watched him walk in the door struggling with the highs and lows of each day. We'd have a conversation filled with details about the exciting new challenges of the workday only to have it end with a sorrowful silence when it came time to discuss the different and most difficult challenge for Jon, losing his dad. Once again I tried to convince Jon that he should at least mention the situation to his new boss. I thought that by Jon admitting the inevitable out loud to someone other than me, perhaps he would begin to deal with it himself.

On January 11, at the age of sixty-three, Jon's father finally gave up his fight. Jon, along with both of his brothers and both of his aunts, stood by his dad's side during his final moments. Witnessing a person take his last breath is just as powerful and moving as watching a newborn take his first breath; Jon had experienced both in a span of just eight months. He came home from the hospital late that night as I paced back and forth, alone with my thoughts after settling all of the kids in for the night. He looked gray and drawn, as if a giant paintbrush had just whitewashed him, blurring the lines between him and his surroundings. I didn't know what to say; I just held him quietly as the tears finally came.

As the girls came down for breakfast the next morning, my eyes filled with tears again as I realized they would need to be told about their beloved Poppy. They understood that he had been sick, but I didn't know if they could comprehend at four years old the finality of death. Jon and I discussed the question of whether or not they should attend the funeral; would they forever wonder where Poppy went if they didn't get to say good-bye? I recalled going to my great-grandmother's funeral at the age of eleven; for years I hadn't been able to shake the disturbing image of her waxen skin against the peach dress she wore and her freshly applied coat of peach nail polish. I felt it was important that Mady and Cara were spared that kind of anguish and instead were allowed to remember their grandfather in a more positive light—as the smiling, gentle man who always had room on his lap and a hug to go with it.

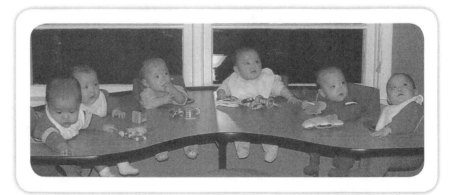

Feeding time!

12 Growing Pains

Even youths grow tired and weary ...
but those who hope in the LORD
    will renew their strength.

Isaiah 40:30 – 31

The year 2005 began with a shadow of sadness lurking in the recesses of our hearts as we mourned the passing of Jon's dad. It was the middle of the cold and dismal days of winter after over a year of difficulties beyond what we ever could have imagined. We felt that God had taken us to the bottom of the deepest ocean. We had two choices: get mired in the muck and drown by dropping the anchor of depression and self-pity, or swim with all the might God gave us, looking to Him, our light and our salvation, to carry us to the surface.

It was a new year, Jon had a new job, and we felt it was time to adopt a new attitude. Jon and I became determined to finally go on the offense instead of merely dodging the challenges and heartbreaks that came our way. A new resolve buried deep beneath the pressing weight of responsibility miraculously began to rise up in me. If someone were to peer in our front window, they would've still seen a house bursting at the seams with eight kids, various volunteers, and two droopy-eyed young parents desperately trying to keep their heads above water. However, if that person could somehow also peek into our hearts, they would see the tiniest shimmer of nervy confidence that said not only were we going to be a family who survived the birth of eight children in less than four years, but we were going to thrive in the warm waves of God's blessings.

The daily routine continued to be almost as strict as boot camp; it had to be to avoid complete mayhem. The house was plastered with lists and reminders — who got which medicine for a cold, how much and at what time, who had a doctor's appointment, which diapers fit which baby and in which drawer of the changing table they were kept, and what day the girls had to take snacks for their class. I even had a list by the changing table for volunteers to check off who pooped that day.

It was interesting how different people viewed my incessant list making. Some viewed it as a serious sign that I was just an obsessive-compulsive control freak. They rolled their eyes as fresh reminders to "wash hands thoroughly" were taped to the bathroom mirror during flu season. Others saw the lists as a huge help, enabling them to know exactly what I needed to make my house run smoothly, therefore resulting in a much happier — and sometimes even slightly quieter — household. Still others didn't seem to see the lists at all. I would hear someone bellowing from the family room, "Kate, where are the diapers?" and for the tenth time that week, I'd answer, "Look on the drawers; they're labeled!"

The girls started to actually enjoy moments with the babies who were getting to be roly-poly enough to be the epitome of squishy baby cuteness! I'm sure Cara and Mady would be quick to emphasize the "moments" part of that statement however, for by the end of each day, the noise level in our house was enough to send even the most gregarious of four-year-olds running.

During the turmoil of December, it became obvious that I had to push the six to the next level; they were not NICU babies anymore. We started to place them in the most valuable piece of furniture in our house at the time, based, of course, on its unparalleled usefulness: the six-seat feeding table. Jon and I purchased the table from a company that makes items for day-care facilities. It looked like a bean shaped table on sturdy narrow legs with six red plastic molded seats inserted along the outside edge of the table.

The first time I placed each baby in his individual seat, I stood back and laughed. They looked like a bunch of little old men and ladies, mostly toothless, hunched over the table. Collin had an especially difficult time holding up his big old head; it was not an easy task. It was obvious that all of them needed to strengthen their core muscles, and distracting them with food while encouraging them to sit sturdily was the perfect solution.

After just the first few feedings of organic baby food were cautiously spooned into their mouths, they became extremely excited about being placed at the table. Usually by mealtime, their medley of shrieking cries could probably be heard from the street, but within minutes, they would all be struggling like baby birds to open their little mouths wide enough to catch every drop. The few minutes of quiet were always a welcome reprieve, but it didn't last long if my spoon lagged for even just a moment. I probably looked like a robotic maniac set on high speed shoveling applesauce into each little mouth as fast as I could. Looking back, it would've been humorous had I had the time or energy to enjoy it.

I found each day an ever-changing series of transitions and adjustments; the babies seemed to be developing and growing by the moment. I tried desperately to take in and appreciate each new milestone, but sadly, it was nearly impossible. I kept my camera at the ready sitting on top of the entertainment center in the family room. I did manage to snap sweet memories here and there, like Alexis's open mouthed, wide eyed, no-holds-barred grin or Leah's spirited little crinkly nose smile, but it just never felt like enough.

One thing that makes me so sad is thinking about all the moments I missed. I was either up in the kitchen or down in the laundry room for at least three quarters of my waking hours. The family room, the

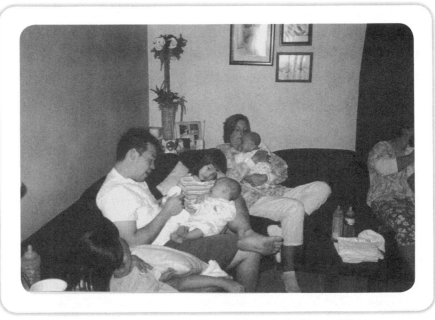

*Mady with screaming Joel, Daddy with Collin and Cara,
and Nurse Angie in the background with Aaden.*

room where the babies spent almost all their time, was on the floor in between my two destinations. About six steps separated each level, and so often I longed to just drop the laundry basket and crawl on the floor with my exploring babies as I passed through the room. Very seldom did I have that luxury. I was on duty, on task. How else would it all get done? I knew that if I slacked off for even just one day, the next day would be twice as demanding. Pressure was my middle name.

A godsend in the form of a capable young night nurse saved us from many sleepless nights. We had filtered through nurses three times for various reasons, and as soon as I met Angie, I knew we had finally found the right fit. She was a mom herself (her two girls were close to Mady and Cara's age) and even more importantly, she exuded calm, easy control. "Not easily flustered" was a primary personality trait for anyone wanting to survive even one day at our house.

With Angie working the night shift from 1:00 a.m. to 9:00 a.m., we were able to establish a better nighttime routine. All six babies were taken up to their individual cribs after their last feeding. The room had long ago been rearranged with all six cribs lining the perimeter of the room, which allowed just enough space for one dresser and one changing table. In an effort to have the babies sleep through the night without being woken by their tired big sisters clomping past their room on their way up to bed, I would turn the overhead fan on low and press the button on their small sound machine on the dresser. Within minutes, as the white noise filled the room, the squawking uprising would quiet — usually. We'd hear sniffles and shuffles on the monitor, signaling that everyone had resigned themselves to blankets and pacifiers until hopefully seven o'clock the next morning.

When our bedtime routine actually became more predictable and Angie eventually switched to day shift three days a week, Jon and I got the courage after a quick dinner one night to declare our Independence Day. I longed to be free from relying on anyone other than my core group of about four volunteers, who by that time were also dear friends, and I pondered aloud the what-ifs of beginning to do the bedtime feedings on our own. As Jon listened, he agreed to give it a try, and I smiled tentatively as I reached for the phone to cancel my volunteers who were scheduled to arrive in less than an hour. The thought of being in my house with just my husband, and the two of us settling all of our children into their beds for the night actually made me giddy. Even better though was the feeling of accomplishment later that night as Jon and I dropped into bed after doing with our four hands what was normally difficult to do with twelve.

That long dreary winter seemed like it would never end. Being in the house almost twenty-four hours a day with eight kids gave a whole new meaning to cabin fever. At that time we still did not have a vehicle large enough to hold our entire family, and I felt slightly imprisoned. It wasn't like I could wake up in the morning, decide I needed some groceries, pack my baby up in the car seat, and set off for the local store. Everything had to be carefully planned around feeding times and volunteer availability because I had to leave the babies at home.

If I felt like I was under house arrest, then so too did the babies and the twins. The babies were confined even further, to the four walls of their little haven in the family room; it was far easier and safer to keep them together, therefore alleviating the need to constantly keep track of who was where.

The winter blues weren't the only menace that we struggled to keep at bay; colds and ear infections were an almost constant battle. More often than not, a cold would go through the half dozen babies in spite of my ambitious attempts to prevent the spread of germs. Often I would need to administer breathing treatments to those babies who had difficulty conquering a nasty cold. Being preemies, any tiny sniffle somehow managed to turn into a shallow breathy wheeze. Alexis was particularly susceptible and needed treatments quite often; however, everyone certainly had his or her turn.

Even more troublesome was the necessity for synergist injections, again, to aid in warding off RSV, a respiratory virus particularly dangerous for preemies. The shots were to be administered once a month between October and April. I had a major problem: how would I get all six babies to a doctor's office once a month without a car that would fit the babies, the twins, and me? Even if I did have a van, how would I get all the babies into the office without the help of at least two volunteers? And even if I made several trips, I would then need the help of more volunteers, some to come with me and some to stay with the babies left behind. Besides all of the above pitfalls, I would also be exposing them to even more germs that lingered in the pediatrician's office during the winter months. I needed a better plan: I would administer the shots myself.

Since I was a nurse, I felt comfortable calculating the correct dosage based on each baby's weight, and the doctor, after double-checking my dosages the first time, also became comfortable with me administering the medicine. While my mind was able to do the math, my heart had a more difficult time. Although I had injected many infants, they were never my own; I had to really talk myself into jabbing my own baby with a needle and then repeating it five more times. The nurse in me won over my mommy sensitivities. I reasoned that if they were going to get stuck, it may as well be from me in the comfort of their own home.

When the dreaded day came to give the first dose, I picked up Leah and swallowed hard as she smiled and jabbered at me. Resting her on the changing table, I had to place a burp cloth over her head for just an instant as I poked the needle into her skin. I hated the thought of her thinking I was causing her pain. Like most babies, Leah howled furiously at the sudden painful pinch, but after a few minutes of being snuggled close to my heart, she quieted enough for me to move on to my next patient. Five more times I swallowed hard as I reminded myself that one injection every thirty days was far better than dealing with RSV.

As my rowdy crew grew more curious and explorative by the day, they took turns going from an Exersaucer to a blanket strewn with toys on the floor to the much-coveted seat in front of their favorite video, Baby Einstein. A volunteer and I would usually place two at a time at each station for maybe fifteen to twenty minutes — or until one or more screeched loud enough to encourage a faster rotation. Of course there was always someone who was not happy with his or her particular position and complained loudly. In our situation, even though the "squeakiest wheel gets the grease," the squeak had to be pretty convincing. I really wanted to try to train them to entertain themselves, knowing that as part of a big family they would need to be fairly self-sufficient.

I just couldn't possibly give them their way the minute they wanted something.

One day as Beth held Aaden, she and I discussed concerns over the extreme boundaries that defined my babies' world. They were quickly edging toward their first birthday, and yet very few of them had experienced even the most ordinary daily activities such as riding in the front of a grocery cart, feeling the soft fur of a family pet, experiencing the lights and sounds of a crowded public place, or even just an unfamiliar living room. They had been out of the house only to go to doctor appointments. I worried aloud that they had to be bored with the view from behind the white gate that stretched across the bottom of the stairs to the family room.

Ironically as much as they lacked outside stimulation, the constant overstimulation inside our house, from so many people in such a small space day after day, left almost everyone irritable and short-tempered.

At some point just about every day, Aaden would become so rigid and high-strung from the noise level, that he would become inconsolable. Beth figured out right from the beginning that Aaden needed quiet and seclusion. During one particularly noisy nighttime feeding back in the summer, tiny little seven-pound Aaden refused to settle down even to seek comfort in his warm bottle. It became almost scary to watch him as his frenzy of shrill, high-pitched screams left him limp and breathless. I stripped him down to his diaper, searching wildly for any physical signs of what might be bothering him. After thirty minutes of pacing, shushing, swaying, and consoling our wailing Aaden in the midst of the ruckus of five other volunteers and five other hungry babies, Beth asked me if she could take Aaden upstairs to the dark living room where she could hold him quietly and rock him.

Not surprisingly I peeked into the living room just five minutes later and Aaden lay snuggled against Beth, soundly sleeping and looking relaxed and placid at last. Apparently his fragile nervous system was just not able to process all of the constant stimulation.

In the tranquility of that moment a very special bond had been formed and Beth became Aaden's best ally and buddy. Three years later, their bond has deepened and Aaden now sees Beth and proudly declares "Two mommies." It works wonders when he's looking for extra hugs — or maybe just an extra cookie. One would think that it would bother me to have my son refer to anyone else in the world as "Mommy," but by this time I am far beyond that. I realized very early on that although I am Mommy in every sense of the word, it sometimes is a true blessing to know my children have a sort of backup, someone to fill the inevitable gap when there simply is not enough of me to go around. I'm delighted that my kids know they are loved by many people; it makes them freely affectionate, doling out and collecting hugs with unabashed childlike fervor.

After Aaden's need for occasional absolute silence became evident, I once again felt helpless and sad. Sad for Aaden because what choice did he have? Even if our small house could magically absorb the unnerving noise, I could not leave babies unattended in different areas of the house. He, along with all seven of his siblings, was destined to have to deal with the chaos — as well as its unlikely counterpart, isolation from the outside world.

One afternoon I couldn't take the crying one more minute. Not only were the babies beginning to teethe, but Aaden had had a particularly difficult day. Beth happened to be on the schedule to help that day, and when she arrived, she immediately sensed my frustration. "Why don't I take Aaden over to my house for a little bit?" Beth asked. Prior to that day, I had received probably dozens of offers, most from people whom I loved and trusted completely, to take a baby out of the house for a few hours. I never before that moment considered it. I was not accustomed, even when I first had the twins, to having my children out of my care. I just needed to know where they were at all times. But that day, somehow it felt right. I had reached a point where I knew it was in Aaden's best interest to have a bit of solace, and a good dose of fresh air couldn't hurt either. I agreed, and after carefully tucking him into his car seat with a cozy blanket, I was almost envious as I watched him being carried out to the car for his big adventure.

Aaden's first visit was a huge success. Beth delivered him safely home before bedtime, and he looked relaxed and content. It was obvious from his bright-eyed expression that he thought his little outing was pretty fun. Beth told me how he at first seemed to revel in the quietness, resting in the calm, soaking it in. We laughed together as she described how funny he was as he warmed up to his surroundings, sitting on the kitchen counter in his car seat, his eyes scanning side to side like he was at a tennis match. The novelty of new surroundings mixed with a healthy dose of relative silence had both soothed his tenseness and fed his natural baby curiosity.

Beth and I knew we were on to something. Aaden's reaction to a fresh environment made it painfully obvious that all six babies had to get out of the house occasionally, both to get a reprieve from their predictable routine and also to experience new stimuli and situations. It became routine for Beth to take one or two babies for several hours to expose them to different surroundings — or in Aaden's case, to give him a break from the crowded and overstimulating clamor that filled our house.

On one memorable occasion, she took Collin and Aaden to the grocery store. Realizing by that point that adjusting to new situations was sometimes overwhelming for my sheltered and routine babies, she knew the lights and sounds of the store could prompt a potential meltdown. And she was right. When Collin was placed in the front of the cart, a familiar perch for most babies, he was petrified. It was obvious that the blatant unfamiliarity of the entire experience was about as surprising as a cold splash of water, and adjusting to life outside his family room world was going to be an interesting process. He froze in a panic, his screams and body language sending clear messages that he was seriously afraid of the hard metal seat in the rolling cart. His dramatic response drove home the fact that the babies would need to be slowly acclimated to life outside a different kind of womb.

Peeling off the shell of protection that had involuntarily grown around my children became a kind of mission for us. We tried to expose them to a variety of outside stimuli, some as simple and natural as the sensation of the wind in their face. Besides the field trips to Beth's house, my sister Kendra would occasionally whisk a baby away for the day—most often Joel. My friend Susan would sometimes offer to take Hannah and Leah. Of course, there were also our steadfast and devoted teachers and helpers, Nanny Joan and Nanna Janet who worked the front lines at home, constantly challenging and nurturing all of the babies. But as I saw how happy my little explorers were after time spent on their mini excursions, I was deeply relieved that spending almost their entire first year in their carpeted quarters had not permanently hindered their social development. I continued to pray each morning for the warmer days of spring to arrive so I could throw open the door of the family room and go out on the deck for a necessary and much anticipated change of scenery for us all.

With the promise of spring still months away, the hour or so between naptime and dinner was the most challenging part of each day. My kids were voracious eaters and loudly let me know when their little bellies were empty. They would all manage to either roll or scootch to get themselves to the white gate, and they would put on a pitiful performance of wailing and shrieking, knowing that I was flying around the tiny kitchen, with pots and pans clanking and oven door slamming. Cara and Mady, skipping around the toy-strewn family room and replacing dropped pacifiers, did an admirable job most days at trying to entertain and distract them long enough for me to prepare their meal. However, it was not an easy task, and the girls, looking forward to dinner themselves, had little tolerance for the maddening medley of cries.

As a reprieve several times a week, Kayla, Beth's second oldest daughter, would walk the six or seven blocks from the high school to hold and entertain the babies while I fixed their dinner. They loved her hands-on approach as she stretched out on the floor and allowed them to crawl all over her—drooling, dribbling, and so happy to have someone on their eye level if even for a short while. Later she could be found sitting at the helm of the red table quickly doling out heaping mouthfuls of green beans and applesauce. It was a luxury on those few afternoons a week to hear at least some of the six of them giggling instead of crying while I served Mady and Cara their dinner at a much less frantic pace.

One highlight of those bleak winter months was when wiry little Joel managed to get up on all fours and crawl. He surprised everyone with his determined approach to snagging a favorite toy with his new-found mobility and independence. Everyone who passed through the room praised his antics, and his silly gummy grin showed he was very proud of his latest accomplishment. It was not very long before most of the others took note and also conquered the art of crawling; all that is, except Alexis.

I had been concerned with both Alexis as well as Collin at one point. They just didn't seem to have the physical coordination of the other four babies. True, they were always among the biggest of the group, and I thought maybe their size somehow made it more difficult to scoot about like their siblings. When he was five and a half months, I noticed that Collin strongly favored his right side, keeping his left fist gripped tightly and immobile. I had him go through physical therapy, and we soon cleared that hurdle with some extra training for those weak and uncooperative muscles. He quickly caught up with the gang and managed to confidently master crawling by ten months.

Alexis though, was purely content to just sit. Not only did she sit, but she had an awkward tripodlike posture with both of her legs spread unusually wide, aided by her substantially padded bottom instead of the strength of her abdominal muscles. Most perplexing was the fact that she remained plopped in one spot, even to the point of being a sitting duck for sly incoming toy thieves like Joel. She'd screech like a wild woman at the injustices she suffered at the hands of her brothers and sisters who quickly learned they could easily pluck a rattle from her hands and make their escape without threat of retaliation. That was not at all congruent with Alexis's larger than life personality; she was a mover and shaker who was not moving and shaking.

Fortunately, like so many of my deepest fear and worries, there was nothing physically wrong with Alexis. I had a few pointers from a physical therapist in how to encourage her to strengthen those muscles that seemed to be a bit weak, but the real issue was that Alexis would do things on her own timetable, not ours.

Spring, glorious spring, finally arrived that year much to everyone's great relief. The golden rays of sunshine streaming in through the open windows lit up the family room where the babies practiced pulling themselves up on just about anything within reach. They were at such a cute age! I loved when their fine downy hair standing on end from static electricity and backlit with the sunlight made them look like they had little halos.

One day in March I marveled with my sister Kendra at how big the babies were growing; such lively, busy little sponges just soaking everything in and changing so much every day. She hesitated for just an instant before looking me square in the eye and emphatically saying, " Kate, we need to get the babies to Grandma and Grandpa's house for a visit, soon." My heart felt so heavy as I saw the sadness in her expression. She was trying to gently explain to me that while I had been in my foggy, groggy, baby-filled hiatus from reality, life had marched steadily onward. For my dear eighty-six-year-old grandpa, that meant the final season of his long, loving life on this earth was drawing to a close.

My maternal grandparents were, in my mind, the epitome of God's unwavering, unconditional love. They lived their full lives freely giving

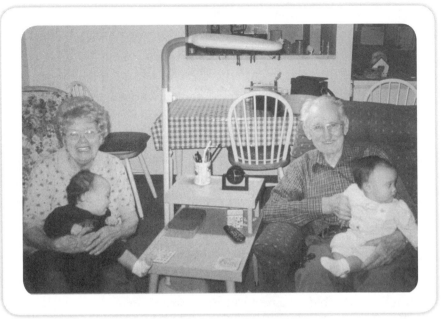

*Grandma holding Joel and Grandpa
holding Hannah, March 2005.*

their heart, their wisdom, and their gifts to anyone who had need, without one string ever being attached. I valued their guidance, grace, and goodness; and although I spoke to them at least a few times a week, I longed for their embrace.

I got Kendra's message loud and clear. I didn't quite know how we were going to pull it off, but I decided right there that we were going for a visit—all of us. At that time, I had not been out of the house with all of the babies at once, except for a very well-planned doctor visit to Hershey, with the help of several volunteers, to get their eyes checked way back in the summer. So it was a *big* deal.

Kendra, Jon, and I put our heads together and came up with a plan. Kendra and her husband, Jeff, would leave their two children with a sitter for the day to allow enough room in their van for four car seats. Jon and I would take our white minivan, also with four kids. It took me every spare minute of an entire day to gather together all of the necessary items required to leave the house for what would amount to a full eight hours.

My biggest concern was Aaden. He had aspiration pneumonia at the time, and although it was not contagious for Grandpa, I worried about taking a sick baby on a two-hour car ride. But time was of the essence.

The look of surprise on Grandma's face when we walked in her front door made it worth every ounce of planning and energy it had taken to get there. She clapped with glee, her gentle eyes twinkling with tears, as she took in the sight of her brood of great-grandchildren, as one by one they were carried in to meet her and Grandpa. My grandparents lived in a tiny assisted living apartment; when the parade of babies finally ended, we stood and laughed at the comically crowded living room. The six little ones all sat in the middle of the room on an outstretched blanket, looking intrigued and yet not quite sure of what to make of this new experience called visiting.

As I looked at my grandfather, I could still see the tender kindness behind the deeply etched lines on his face and his hazy elderly gaze. Sadly though, he looked thin and painfully weak and frail. I knew of no one who had more heart than my grandpa, but I also knew that heart—as in guts, conviction, faith, discipline, and discernment—although honorable, could not change the fact that our physical heart would one day grow old and tired. And that's what was happening with Grandpa.

I gently lifted ten-month-old Hannah onto his bony lap. As she studied her great-grandpa with big dark eyes, he stroked her soft silky hair with his veined hand. With a shaky voice he whispered to Hannah, "You have such beautiful hair, sweetheart." Thankfully, as babies always somehow do, Hannah seemed to sense the genuine love in her old grandpa's heart, and she sat patiently for several minutes before Grandpa lost his strength and gave her up to her daddy. I knew in that instant that my dear grandpa had already begun the transition from this world to the next, because at no time ever in his life had he surrendered the warm, tender embrace of a baby so willingly.

Meanwhile, Grandma, my breath of fresh air, continually thanked us over and over again for making the trek to their house. She was as excited as a child on Christmas morning, and her energy was purely contagious. With her bright eyes locked on our always-engaging baby Alexis, she exclaimed loudly, "Oh, Art, now when we close our eyes, we can see!" It was her own way of saying we were always in her thoughts, another gift unknowingly placed in my heart.

In Grandma's presence I knew how it felt to live in the shelter of kindness and acceptance. I knew since childhood, having grown up with very stringent guidelines and rules, that nothing could ever separate me from her loving embrace. That day was a sweet reminder of how much I longed to be a conduit of that kind of love for my children, just as Grandma always was for me.

Jon also had a special bond with my grandma. Being night owls, both of them spent many late night hours on the phone since we were first married. Jon valued her wisdom and marveled at her knowledge of the Bible. She would relate specific stories to him in vivid detail and then give him chapter and verse so he could check it out for himself if he wanted. Grandma didn't just preach God's Word; she lived and breathed it.

Sadly, that would be the only visit my kids had with their great-grandparents. Grandpa succumbed to congestive heart failure on a hot, humid day in June 2005, and Grandma went on to join him a little more than one year later in September 2006. On days when I really wish I could just talk to them one more time, all I can do instead is pray that someday I will grow up to be just like them. To this day when I am having a bad day, I can still hear Grandpa's voice saying, "You are doing a great job, honey. Keep it up!"

Back at home, the excitement of our big outing had worn off minutes after carrying eight sleeping kids into the darkened house. Jon and I instantly slipped back into action. Teething was in full swing and quickly taking its toll on all of us. It was routine for me to give every one of them a dose of Motrin after their bath at night. We went through innumerable bottles of the syrupy medicine; it was truly a life-saver when dealing with sometimes several babies getting several teeth for several weeks at a time.

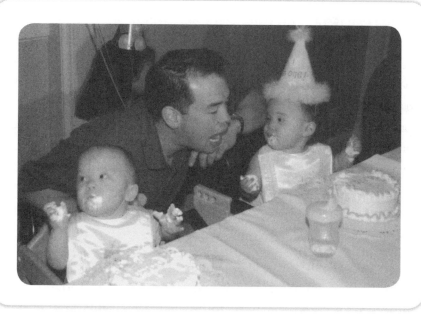

Aaden, Daddy, and Hannah at the babies'
first birthday party.

Speaking of bath time, that was always Jon's specialty. After being away from the house and kids essentially the entire day, this was his time to reconnect with each of them. After dinner while I did kitchen cleanup duty—blessedly alone—he would carry them upstairs and plop them behind the gate that kept them safely contained in their bedroom. He'd strip everybody down to his or her diaper and then walk across the hall to start the water. Six little nearly naked squirming and squealing babies was comical and entertaining, as each of them loved the freedom from clothes, onesies, and especially socks. I'd smile to myself as I'd hear them clamoring at the gate, knowing their favorite time of the day awaited them.

After they were brought downstairs, freshly lotioned and wearing cozy pj's, they would have their final bottle of the night. Meanwhile, Cara and Mady took their turn in the small bathroom, singing and splashing in the shower while Daddy waited patiently with yet another set of fluffy towels and pink pajamas. The whole process took at least an hour, and I always looked at it as a gift from Jon.

I don't know of many dads who would willingly come home from a full workday after an hour and a half commute each way and still take on the energetic and all-consuming task of bathing eight children. And this was not something he did once in a while; this was something he did nearly every single night. Some women get jewelry, fancy gifts, or expensive dinners when their husband wants to get in their good graces. Not me. Give me a man who allows me a solid hour by myself while he manages to wash sixteen sticky hands and eight goopy noses, wrestle all those pudgy damp limbs into pajamas, and then follow it all up with eight individual hugs. I'm pretty sure I got the best of the best when God handed out gifts.

As the monumental marker of the babies' first birthday quickly approached, Jon and I decided to host a huge celebration. We considered it a birthday/thank-you/survival party. We had much to be grateful for during that first year, and so many people to thank. Also, we considered it a major milestone to have actually survived an entire year that consisted of approximately thirteen thousand diaper changes, almost as many bottle feedings, and nearly one thousand loads of laundry. Throw in two highly emotional deaths up to that point, the loss of two jobs, and absolutely zero personal space and privacy, and—well, if surviving all that isn't cause for celebration, I don't know what is.

I furiously planned for months every detail of the big event that would be held at the Inn at Reading, a local venue that could comfortably serve the one hundred guests we expected to attend. It gave me great pleasure to order sweet little "My First Birthday" hats, each topped with a festive white pom-pom. I even splurged on six white satin bibs that I had embroidered with each child's name. I remember hesitating about spending the extra money, but I knew even then, thanks to the whirlwind of that first year, that I had to grab every opportunity I could to capture each fleeting memory. Those tiny bibs now carry sweet nostalgia as I look back on those complicated, crazy, miracle-filled days — and that is worth more than any money can buy.

When the big day arrived, we still didn't have a van large enough to transport everyone at once, so even for their thank-you party, volunteers had to help get us there. We arrived at the Inn, and after about thirty minutes of shuttling the babies, the twins, the diaper bags, and other assorted party paraphernalia into the large dining space, we looked around — and gasped. It was astounding to see everyone who had actually had a hand in helping us in some way in one place. Everywhere I looked were round tables filled with smiling friends, family, and business representatives who just came to say an "Amen" to a job well done by all. If it's true, as the saying goes, that "it takes a village to raise a child," then surely we were looking at six villages represented in that room, who had all worked together with one heart and one purpose to bless our six wide-eyed miracles — as well as our entire family.

Jon and I had arranged for a large, long table to be placed at the front of the room where we could comfortably seat all eight kids. After a nice buffet-style meal, several waitresses placed six small individual birthday cakes, one in front of each baby, all iced in soft pastel colors and decorated with each baby's name. It felt like the entire room held its collective breath as we waited to see who would be the first to discover that wonderful taste of childhood — sugar! With so much to look at, I honestly can't recall who dove in first, but I can say this: after the first few tentative swipes at that tasty icing, news spread fast, and within minutes all six one-year-olds had faces smeared with a rainbow of colors.

I was proud of Cara and Mady as they managed quite nicely to deal with all the attention the babies received, not only on that day but every day. Sometimes I think they relinquished their entire toddlerhoods as the flood of baby talk, baby worries, baby duties, and finally baby milestones washed over every area of our lives. I longed to protect them, and yet, I knew that as the older sisters of sextuplets they were destined for a life far different from the ones Jon and I had envisioned for them. They would need to share their parents, their toys, their snacks—and the spotlight as well.

The party ended on a happy note as we packed up our entourage and headed for home. We knew that the celebration had not been solely the culmination of the first blurry year, but more so the starting point of a whole new set of challenges. Many unknowns and questions hovered just out of sight. People would ask questions like, "How are you all fitting in that house? Did you find a van yet? Can you imagine when they are all sixteen? What about college?" People must not have realized that I would end up in the loony bin if I concentrated on those questions. Of course Jon and I worried about and discussed each and every one of those issues and a hundred more, but we also knew that we could not allow fear to get a foothold in our life and therefore steal the joy that all eight of our children brought to us every day.

We went back to our little house on Dauphin Avenue that afternoon more determined than ever to take one day at a time while using the knowledge and wisdom we gathered along the way to forge plans for what would no doubt be an exciting future.

Officially graduating to one-year-old status in our house meant that bottles would become a thing of the past. Just as I had with the girls, I decided to introduce milk in a cup at mealtimes. As with most new stages, one or two would lag behind; in this case, it was Aaden and Joel. They could have a cup, but they had to remain on formula until they managed to surpass at least the tenth percentile on the doctor's growth chart. I tried and tried, but fattening up those two boys seemed nearly impossible.

The babies took to their "cuppies" fairly easily, and within weeks we bid farewell to one more icon of infancy. The picture of an eighteen pound, twenty-six-inch-tall peanut fiercely clutching a seemingly huge sippee cup was hilarious, but I was so happy to be free of bottle duty.

Aaden's lack of body fat, while putting him in the back of the line for milk, only seemed to work in his favor in the "who would walk first" category. Just days after his May tenth birthday, the little stinker teetered and tottered on his scrawny legs, one hesitant step, and then two. On the other end of the scale, Hannah, definitely neck and neck with Collin for leading the pack in size, proved my smaller-babies-will-walk-first theory completely wrong as she went toe to toe with Aaden, taking her first few steps right along with him.

When Nanny Joan popped in for a visit later that day, she good-naturedly set her "Little Lovely Leah" on her lap for a heart-to-heart about walking. We laughed as Leah crinkled up her nose, loving the animated chitchat with her favorite visitor. We laughed even harder though when just days later, Leah made her Nanny Joan proud by showing off her delicate little tiptoe-y steps, two or three at a time. Raucous applause erupted all around as we all hooted and hollered, hoping to encourage Joel, Collin, and Alexis to give it a try also.

They, however, were not impressed. Joel was content with his title as "fastest crawler" and didn't see much use in complicating his mode of transportation at all. It was about that time when Joel went from speed demon, daredevil, toy-swiping cruiser to the head-bopping target for the two-legged travelers. They now had an advantage with their higher perspective, and they'd innocently — or maybe not — hit him on the head with whatever toy they carried as they passed him by. Poor Joel. He did eventually see the wisdom in stepping up to the challenge, literally, and after months of whining, finally got up the nerve to walk!

Collin—well, I'm going to have to say it again—the poor little guy had his head to contend with. Every time it seemed he gained his balance and might just take a step or two, the weight of his head would make him topple. It was somewhat comical, and yet a bit sad. Thankfully Collin's stubborn determination eventually paid off, and he, too, caught up with the crowd within a few months.

Alexis would be on her own timetable in life. She was either joyful and goofy, flashing her huge open-mouth grin with that mischievous twinkle in her eye, or she was like a screech owl, letting loose with a shriek that made my ears ring at times. There was no middle ground. True to form, there really wasn't much middle ground when it came to moving her bottom either. She had already made it clear that she was not big on the whole idea of crawling. After all, there were plenty of people around, most often Mady or Cara, who were quite efficient at delivering a desired toy at the beginning of the screechiest crescendo. Her system was working, and she knew it. On the other hand, at seventeen and a half months old, I worried again that something might be physically causing her delay. My pediatrician assured me she was still in the "normal" range and that, especially for a preemie, she was doing just fine. I really wasn't convinced—until one wonderful day when sedentary Alexis decided she was ready to take a new stance and finally took her first few steps. Yeah!

They now had all officially graduated to toddlers. Oh my heavens . . .

With the increased mobility inside our house, it became more painfully obvious that our lack of mobility outside the house, namely a van, was a serious issue. It was no longer bitterly cold outside. The flowers were blooming, the warmth of the summer sun was uplifting, and the kids and I were just aching to escape our monotonous daily routine. I found myself daydreaming of Jon and I taking the kids for a leisurely Sunday drive, a seemingly simple event that we had never done with all of our children.

Jon began the earnest search for the most suitable vehicle that would meet all of our specific requirements. We needed it to be large enough to comfortably fit eight car seats and two adults, plus have cargo space that would hold two triple strollers. It had to be reliable and get good gas mileage. A huge bonus, as Jon pointed out, would be to have enough head room to stand as we lifted babies in and out of car seats.

It was not an easy bill to fill, but after diligently researching the ten-passenger van, Jon learned that the Dodge Sprinter met or exceeded every single item on our punch list, even the headroom. I wanted to see for myself if the van would work for us. I knew that if we took the giant leap and purchased the van, then it absolutely had to be a smart investment. We had a lot riding on our investment, no pun intended, and could not afford to buy a headache.

Our local Dodge dealership, Savage, was extremely accommodating and brought the Sprinter to our house on a warm July afternoon for a test drive. As it pulled into the driveway, I got very nervous. It was huge. I wondered how I would ever be able to maneuver that ungainly monster in a parking lot. But I saw the sparkle of excitement in Jon's eyes as he checked off every last requirement on our list. He knew how to get to me—the list—and I could not deny that the "Big Blue Bus," as it later came to be known, would indeed serve us well and become our ticket to finally being able to get out of the house. Ferrying eight kids, diaper bags, strollers, and snacks to the van would not be easy, but at least it would now be possible.

The experienced salesman covered all his bases, bringing the appropriate papers with him to the house that night. After a short discussion, Jon and I made our decision. With Jon's Jeep traded in as the down payment, we became the proud new owners of a navy blue 2004 Dodge Sprinter.

Mady and Cara were jumping up and down in the driveway. We had promised them a ride in the new van that very night if everything went as planned. Getting an energy boost from their overflowing excitement,

I followed them back into the house to begin packing everyone up for our very first jaunt as a family of ten.

I changed all of the babies into their pajamas as Cara and Mady scrambled into theirs. Jon worked up a sweat with the tedious task of tethering all eight car seat bases into the van; after nearly a full hour of scurrying around, we were all strapped in and ready to go.

Wanting to share our excitement, we set off down the boulevard toward Nanny Joan and her husband, Terry's, house. I have to admit, at first I felt somewhat ridiculous. My seat felt like it was five feet off the ground and I almost felt like ducking my head as the top of the van barely seemed to clear some of the lower branches on the tree-lined streets of Wyomissing. Then I peeked back at my sleepy crew. Every one of them sat quietly and curiously looking out the low windows. It was one of those moments I will never forget. Who would have ever imagined that every available seat in a ten-passenger van would hold a member of my precious family? I didn't know whether to laugh or cry. Even today the sight of our loaded "Big Blue Bus" still brings tears to my eyes at times. I am so thankful for our reliable, comfortable, giant box on wheels, but I am even more grateful for the sixteen little pairs of feet dangling over the edge of the car seats on the way to our next adventure.

The new independence I felt by having transportation was coupled with a scarier type of independence when Angie was unceremoniously pulled from her part-time nursing position in my home after working with me for almost a full year. Abrupt as it was—she took a phone call one Friday afternoon at our house, stood up from the table, and was done—it definitely came as no surprise to me, or Angie for that matter. Medicaid had been willing to pay for Angie's services for six months. When the six-month mark came, I knew I could not adequately take care of the many pressing needs of six babies at one time by myself. Joan or Janet or Beth would often help out, and as helpful as that was, it wasn't enough. The dailies, the little things that absolutely had to be done every day, were overwhelming. I relied heavily on Angie's reliable time slots to maintain my footing. And so I decided to fight for six additional months.

I stood my ground by reminding the insurance review board that the law for the ratio between the number of babies and caregivers in a Pennsylvania day care facility was just 3:1. How could it be safe for me to take care of not only six one-year-olds but also two four-year-olds? On a good day, I managed it—though it was hectic and hairy. However, those days were few and far between as there were many more days when someone had an ear infection, another needed a breathing treatment, someone else bit her brother, and the fourth was vomiting—all with the chirping chorus of "Mommy, I'm hungry" from the big girls in the background. Not to mention all the near misses like when Collin turned blue at the table after nearly aspirating his spoonful of food or when Joel tried to pull himself up but toppled over with his face narrowly missing the edge of the entertainment center. It just wasn't a job that one person, with only two eyes, two hands, and two legs, could safely do by herself for twelve hours every day.

I heard much criticism through the grapevine for my persistent stance. I think there were some people who felt Jon and I had our hand out, always wanting more and more help. Some had the opinion that I had asked for all these babies and it was now my responsibility to care for them, that it should not be my insurance company's burden. I guess in a sense that is exactly why I decided to write this book. I not only want to share the story of our amazing, unusual, unplanned, and unexpected blessings, but I also want to say that I absolutely appreciate more than anyone could imagine every single ounce of help that anyone has ever given in any way. Also, Jon and I have the awesome responsibility of raising our eight children, but we were not called to be martyrs, stupidly neglecting assistance that directly affected the well-being and safety of our children. In everything we did—and do—Jon and I simply wanted to give our kids a fighting chance to lead a somewhat normal life in the most abnormal circumstances.

One day in August of 2005, Jon received an email he thought I should read. Knowing I was far from computer savvy and hated the idea of hunching over his computer to read things, he printed it out and brought it into the kitchen. It was from a television production company that had heard of our family and was interested in doing a one-hour documentary of our story.

"Whoa," I said. "Seriously?"

Jon and I kind of looked at each other. This was not the first time we were approached by the media. It was becoming more and more difficult to duck into the shadows. How did our quiet little existence in the suburbs of Pennsylvania somehow blossom (or maybe *explode* is a better word) into a "story" that someone wanted to tell on national television?

As we discussed our feelings over that sort of exposure for our family, Jon instantly said, "No way!" He felt somewhat vulnerable after having certain information quoted incorrectly, both on television as well as in newspapers, following the firestorm of media that surrounded the birth of the babies. Also, we had experienced firsthand the stress involved with the filming of the makeover on our house. We knew very well that filming anything when it involved eight kids, plus the additional daily upheaval of camera crews squeezed into our already crammed house, would be a definite challenge.

I, however, was always lamenting the fact that with our days being as full as they were, we rarely got the chance to videotape the sweet baby memories and milestones that happened each and every day. I was thrilled with myself when I occasionally managed to grab my tired old camera to quickly capture a funny grin peeking beneath a lopsided hat or a shy peek-a-boo from under a favorite blanket. I knew that someday I would be even sadder when I realized that my kids had passed through a stage so quickly that the only memory I escaped with was that of me holding on for dear life. I loved the thought that a compact hour-long, clipped, cut, edited, story-formatted version of the next six to nine months of the babies lives would be forever available to me at my fingertips. I pictured all ten of us someday sitting down with a big bowl of popcorn, oohing and aahing over how tiny and cute they were. I knew Mady and Cara would also value those memories as they, too, had been whisked through various stages in the whirlwind of our hectic lives.

As I poured out my thoughts to Jon, we decided it couldn't hurt to at least speak with the head of the production company, hopefully to get a better idea of what a "documentary" entailed and then go from there.

Our conversation lasted a full two hours. I carefully and explicitly explained our reservations. We asked question after question and listened very carefully for any signs that filming our children would put them at risk in any possible way. In the end, it was one comment that persuaded both Jon and me to accept the invitation: "We do television to help people understand other people better." It hit a nerve, and I instantly felt a jolt of excitement; this was our opportunity to finally relate to the public our thoughts, hopes, and dreams for our children, while at the same time visually sharing the endearing, yet overwhelming, everyday reality of our situation.

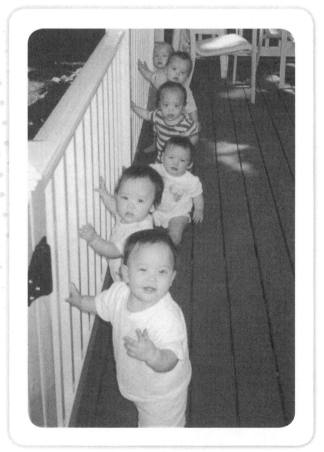

Summer fun, 2005.

13 On the Move

Now to him who is able to do immeasurably more
than all we ask or imagine, according to his power
that is at work within us.

Ephesians 3:20

It was early December and I rushed around the house preparing a
quick dinner for the kids, jotting down last minute instructions
for Joan and Terry who were babysitting the babies, and praying that
I would have enough time to dry my hair. I was nervous but elated
because Jon and I were going out for the night for his first annual
Christmas party held at the Governor's Mansion.

Thinking that six nineteen-month-olds would be more than enough
to keep Joan and Terry busy for the night, the plan was that I would
take Cara and Mady with me and drop them off at Aunt Jodi's and
Uncle Kevin's house in central Pennsylvania. I was to meet Jon there
where he would get freshened up for the night without having to drive
all the way home from Harrisburg to Wyomissing.

I was so excited about the night, anticipating Jon's face when he saw me
in a red beaded skirt instead of my usual household uniform of comfortable sweatpants and a T-shirt. Admittedly I was equally excited about the
idea of a delicious sit-down dinner and adult conversation, and I smiled to
myself as the girls and I pulled into my brother's quiet development.

Almost immediately I noticed a "For Sale" sign to my right in front of
a welcoming brick Cape-style house set in the middle of a wide expanse
of front and back yards. Jon and I had been debating for weeks over what

to do about our crowded living conditions. We had come to the conclusion that we had to do something—and soon. It felt like the walls of our little house in Wyomissing were bulging out, reminding me of pictures I had seen one time of a house hit by a tornado, threatening at any moment to explode from the pressure within. Ironically, at the same time, I also felt like the walls were caving in on me, collapsing all around me as I tripped daily over toys and toddlers. With those cramped reminders, my curiosity was newly piqued, and minutes later as I walked into Kevin and Jodi's kitchen, I was jabbering on and on about how cute the house was and whether or not it could possibly work for our family of ten.

Weighing the pros and cons, I almost dismissed the house, because from the outside it appeared to be not much larger than where we already lived. However, the location was perfect. It would significantly shorten Jon's hour and a half drive to and from work, which would in turn result in much needed relief on our tight budget that was being squelched under the skyrocketing gas prices. More importantly, it was near my brother and his growing family.

We quickly discovered that I indirectly knew the daughter of the owners through childhood connections, so Jon and I decided to at least go and take a look at the interior of the house. I can't even explain how my emotions vacillated when we walked through that front door. I shivered as I somehow realized that I had just turned the page to another new chapter of our lives. I absolutely loved my little house where we had smiled, cried, struggled, and rejoiced since Madelyn and Cara were just eleven months old, but it was time to move on. Standing in the open spaces of the living room and kitchen of this house, I began to see with new eyes what God had laid at our feet.

The house felt airy and uncomplicated. There were several changes I would want to make, mainly replacing the existing carpeting with hardwood flooring, but I could see immediately that it was a house that would be easily maintained. Its simplicity greatly appealed to me. I didn't need expensive bells and whistles in the form of fancy lighting or appliances. I was primarily looking for space—space for our energetic toddlers to run, space for a large dining table, storage space, bedroom space, and closet space.

Traditionally the upper level of a standard Cape-style house is known to have several small bedrooms. In this case however, as we climbed the stairs to the second floor, we saw that the owners had split the entire top level of the house into just two very large bedrooms. It had a full bathroom in the hallway, two exceptionally roomy walk-in closets, and two

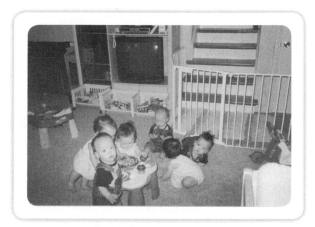

Playtime, summer 2005.

attics spaces. Jon and I knew at first glance that the huge long open layout of the first bedroom was perfect for six cribs while the other brightly lit bedroom worked equally well for the big girls. It was a rather unusual layout that happened to work absolutely perfectly for us.

The layout of the house met other criteria on our long laundry list of necessities as well. For instance, the master bedroom was on the first floor, and the immaculately clean and spacious laundry room was positioned practically right in the center of the first floor between the master bedroom and the kitchen. What a relief it would be to not have to lug full laundry baskets down to the dreary basement, running up and down the stairs ten times a day to hurriedly change loads. We loved the generous flat yard of grass that stretched out behind the house. It could easily hold our swing set and still have more than ample room for eight kids to run and play.

It was an odd ride home after our initial tour of the house. It was one of those times when I was not quite sure if I should laugh or cry. God had answered our prayer by supplying a house for us that met our every need, and yet our sadness hung heavy in the cold air of the car. We both felt strongly that we had found the house for us, and we enthusiastically spewed ideas of where things would fit and how to make it work—only to settle into a silence as each of us absorbed our own thoughts of yet another major life change.

We put our house in Wyomissing on the market that December. Joan convinced me to consider listing it with a company that relies heavily on the seller's participation and therefore charges a fee of only 1.5 percent as opposed to the customary 6 percent on the sale of a home. Initially I dragged my feet, thinking it would be crazy of me to take on such a major project in the midst of a bustling household full of kids. The thought of saving a considerable amount of money in realtor's fees and therefore having a larger down payment toward the new house, however, won me over.

Sundays were designated open house days. Ugh. Every Sunday. It still makes my head spin. Every week Jon and I planned who would take the kids somewhere—they obviously needed to be out of the house for nearly the entire day—and which one of us would stay at the house to greet potential buyers. I pulled out all the stops, cleaning the house from top to bottom, trying my best to declutter every closet and surface. I'd bake chocolate chip cookies, with the help of some quick refrigerated dough; and while the yummy smell wafted throughout the house, I'd scramble to change diapers, wipe faces, tie shoes, smooth down hair, and bundle everyone up in winter coats and hats. After a quick prayer with Jon, I'd light a few candles, scan over my list for anything I'd missed, and race out the door to my vanload of expectant passengers.

Our Sunday adventures varied. For the very first open house I stayed back at the house with Jon while Beth watched the kids at her house for the afternoon. Once we knew what to expect though, I knew Jon could handle showing the house by himself, and my job was to figure out what to do with eight kids for four hours.

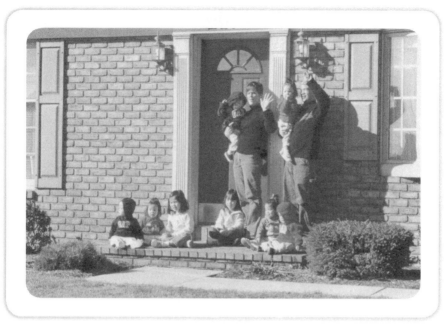

Hello, new house!

One Sunday, Beth's daughter, Kayla, and I decided to brave the local mall with our two triple strollers. I'm sure we looked somewhat comical as people stared at the rolling mountain of babies, coats, and diaper bags. We simply couldn't travel lightly, and we were never able to be inconspicuous. I still struggle with standing out at times. It feels unnatural to be approached by random strangers all with an awed look of disbelief etched on their faces, and their hands outstretched to caress my kids. I know at times I am downright unapproachable, but believe me, it is exhausting to constantly feel like an exhibit at the local zoo, with everyone who passes wanting to reach out and pet your babies.

The following week, looking for a more laid-back afternoon, the kids and I piled into the car and drove the short distance to Nanna Janet's house for a visit. God bless her. It is not just anyone who happily opens her door to a clamorous crew of kids and one very tired and stressed out mommy. The kids loved getting out of the house and exploring new surroundings, so the afternoon was actually a welcome reprieve from our ordinary routine. Several hours later, the Big Blue Bus was blissfully silent as we pulled into our driveway to see if Daddy had sold our house.

My stomach was jittery with nerves as I tried to get a head start on packing. My daily goal was to complete two boxes during nap-time. I tried hard not to allow myself time to reminisce about all the firsts that our little house held. Looking forward took discipline and determination, along with a heaping helping of faith — Jon and I had already purchased our new house in rural Pennsylvania. We had pushed the closing date out as far as possible hoping for a quick sale of our home, but the day was fast approaching when I would need to turn in the paperwork for a swing loan if the sale didn't happen.

Thirty-six days after our house was listed, it sold. We were elated and relieved, and I prayed I would have the necessary energy to begin the serious task of packing up the rest of the house.

●

We had just a few weeks before we closed on the new house to hire con-tractors to freshen up the paint and lay the new hardwood floors before we moved in. Jon was momentarily tempted to lighten our load by just living with the tired old carpeting and paint. However, I felt strongly that if we didn't push to make the house more kid friendly before we got there, we would certainly never have the time to do it all after we got there.

As moving day approached, our small living room was piled high with boxes. I felt like a squirrel stockpiling all my goodies. Every chance I had I would quickly grab a box, fill it, tape it, label it, and stack it. The scary part was that as many items as I seemed to drag out of the closets, base-ment, and remote areas of the house, I'd turn around and realize that I hadn't even begun to touch rooms like the kitchen and babies' room.

With all six toddlers hanging at the white gate, constantly needing either a diaper change, a meal, some mommy-time, or a referee, I knew I wasn't going to be able to pack our most used items and still see to everyone's daily needs. Jon and I agreed that although I was making some headway with one or two boxes at a time, it would eventually come down to a major cram session for the entire week of our impending closing. In order to make that possible, I divided the babies into groups. Beth took Leah, Aaden, and Collin. Kendra took Joel. Janet took Alexis and Hannah. The big girls went to my friend Jamie's house in Michigan. It was a planning nightmare, but I felt relieved to know that they would all be loved and cared for while also being spared the stress and inevitable upheaval that seemed to be stacking up as high as our pile of boxes.

With all the kids out of the house, I went into overdrive. Practically running around the first floor, I started attacking my packing with almost reckless abandon. I knew it would take every ounce of my strength and every last minute we had to collect years of belongings and memories and load them into the three large trucks Jon had rented.

Jon had called two brothers-in-law who in turn called a few friends to lend a hand with the larger items, and while the guys carried load after load out to the waiting trucks, I continued to work my way through the contents of each room. I then turned my attention to scouring and scrubbing each floor, countertop, and bathroom, determined to leave the house, a part of our hearts and history, tidy and as fresh smelling as possible to meet its new owners.

After two eighteen-hour days, Jon and I walked out our front door for the last time. I willed myself to not even look back as I trod down the front walkway. I knew there was no value in pining away over "housie" as the kids called it; I needed to look forward to our future where surely new adventures awaited.

As I held the handle of the van, I hesitated. I suddenly remembered one more thing that I desperately wanted to take from our little house on Dauphin Avenue: several of my grandmother's lilies from the front garden bed. It was dark and chilly and the ground had not completely thawed from its winter slumber, but I had to have just a few. Red eyed and disheveled after a torturous forty-eight hours, Jon carefully dug up a few nuggets of my past and placed them in my hands. We drove away that night as I clutched the lilies, knowing that soon they would be replanted and once again bloom with new life and the promise of sunny days ahead.

14 One Day at a Time

"My grace is sufficient for you, for my power is made perfect in weakness."

2 Corinthians 12:9

I'll say it again: Like most little girls, I had dreamed of the day when I would meet my husband, have children, and settle down to live a happily-ever-after kind of life. Over the past several years, those heart-felt yearnings of my childhood have felt like an eight-fold love note from the Lord tucked in the depths of my soul. He knew my heart, and every good and perfect gift came from Him. I often dug down deep, took out that well-worn promise, and soaked in the goodness of it all. At other times however, that same love note seemed to have been torn in pieces and scattered in the wind, leaving me reeling, sapped of all my strength and vigor while the scraps of what once was my life rained down around me.

Having twins and then sextuplets was never in my childhood dreams; and yet that is the destiny God has chosen for me. Meeting Jon, getting married, and having the girls seemed to fit perfectly with what I had imagined. The "happily-ever-after part" seemed to be lost forever in a sea of six little blips on an ultrasound screen. In time, however, devastation, fear, and anger turned to resignation, acknowledgment, and acceptance. I wanted more than acceptance, though. I knew accepting the fate I had been dealt was just the first step. I wanted to not only survive my calling; I wanted to rise up, grasp it with both hands, and *thrive* in my calling as Jon's wife and the mother of all eight of our children.

The only way to do that was to pay close attention to the lessons God was teaching me. While I could possibly list a hundred such lessons, I will, in honor of our six life-changing miracles, limit my list to just the following six:

1. God is in control

Since the moment Jon and I discovered I was pregnant with sextuplets, we could maintain our sanity only because we knew that God is in control. One of my favorite Scriptures is Romans 8:28: "And we know that in all things God works for the good of those who love him, who have been called according to his purpose." At first, I found the "all things" part a little hard to believe. I wanted to ask God if He was sure He didn't mean "most things." As much as I wanted to believe Him, I continually ran down my list of "buts" for God, just in case He had forgotten. "But God," I would begin, "what about what the doctors said? That the chances of my babies all surviving are minuscule? That I could possibly die? What about the fact that You have only given me two hands, Lord, to care for six babies? And we have a small house, remember, Lord. Oh, and Jon has no job, Lord. How will we provide for our children?" My rantings went on and on until finally I knew I needed to turn my whining and questioning completely inside out. In spite of all the grim statistics and the mental, physical, and logistical challenges, I learned that when "but God" popped into my mind, that instead of falling into the pit of doubt and despair, I needed to attach a new ending to my thought: But God ... is in control—and that meant that He would indeed work together *all* things for my good!

I can't say this revelation came easily to me. I am one of those people who cherishes being in control at all times. To completely trust God and relinquish my control is an ongoing struggle. Every time I feel things are going well in my life, I find myself once again tempted to take back the reins. Several times in the last few years, especially, the Lord allowed me to do just that. I'd think to myself, "I can do this. My days are falling into place, all my ducks are in a row"—which usually meant the kids were napping, I had only one more load of laundry to dry, and dinner was smelling great in the oven — and then it would happen. Two kids would wake up with the flu — so much for my last load of laundry. Dinner smoldered in the oven as I cleaned up, and I felt utterly ineffective and, yes, out of control.

It took me many months to realize that it is during those times in my life when I am feeling utterly out of control that I can actually do what God has called me to do all along; that is, rely on Him. He is a big God who knows all of my human limitations and failures and He does not allow one aspect of my life to fall through the cracks or be overlooked. By allowing Him to lead the way and take control, I can trust that the responsibility of "all things" will no longer weigh me down.

2. God is gracious and strong

Back when I was on bed rest, feeling weak and irritable, I had in a sense, hit rock bottom. Not only was I not in control, I realized that without God's grace and strength to carry me through those days, I simply would not make it. Isaiah 40:31 reminded me that, "those who hope in the LORD will renew their strength. They will soar on wings like eagles; they will run and not grow weary, they will walk and not be faint."

It would be ridiculous to say that God in His infinite goodness and grace has delivered me into a land where endless diaper changes, meals, laundry piles, teething, toddling, and tattling has no effect on *my* measure of grace and energy. The good news is that I have learned that when I run out of grace and energy, God, if I just stand out of His way long enough, is always there with a fresh supply for me to tap into. His well is never empty, and He is always gracious enough to give me the strength for each new day. As He did during my pregnancy especially, He'll simply reach down, scoop me up, and carry me. Gracious and strong, He's a good God!

3. God can be trusted

When Jon and I walked bleary-eyed around our house, each of us holding two infants while still two more waited their turn, I couldn't see beyond that particular moment. If I allowed myself to pan out for a broader view of our precarious situation, I quickly would feel my fight or flight instinct take effect. Fortunately, as many times as I was tempted to just run away, God began to teach me how to trust in Him instead.

He knew our finances were quickly running dry. He knew that as much as I needed Jon's two capable arms helping me through each day, that he, on the other hand, needed to find a job that would provide some personal satisfaction as well as dig us out of our financial quandary. He also knew that as a literal thinker, I was going to need concrete lessons in trust as I learned to rely completely on His provision.

In order for me to learn to trust, I first needed to learn how to hear God's voice and obey. One such opportunity came to me through a story my sister Kendra shared with me. She told me about a family in her church who had struggled through the Christmas season due to the father being unemployed. I remember thinking, "Ugh. Been there, done that," and my heart went out to them. However, I didn't think I could possibly help; I had eight kids of my own to feed. And then I heard it, that still small voice. It was saying that in the midst of so many kindnesses shown to me that I needed also to be sensitive to the needs of others around me. I admit that at first I buried that voice as quickly as I could under my long, personal list of financial worries. I asked God how He could possibly ask me to give away to complete strangers what very little we had at the time; and still He persisted.

God, I learned is not only persistent but He is tireless. After dodging God for days, a lightbulb finally went on — God was looking for obedience from me. I whipped out my checkbook and with a cheerful yet somewhat doubtful attitude I scribbled in an amount and marched it immediately out to the mailbox. Standing in the cold and looking into my mailbox, I hastily shoved the envelope in — and was pleasantly surprised to see a small envelope with a bright Christmas bow on it. As I walked back up the driveway I tore it open and almost sank to my knees. I held in my hand a gift card from a neighbor I barely knew for the exact amount that I had just written on my check. Some of you are thinking, "Big deal. It was just a coincidence." I don't believe in coincidence, and I knew God had just taught me something big. He proved to me that I would never be able to out-give Him. He would always know my exact needs. My only job was to trust and obey.

4. God is love

"Mommy, can you fill my cuppy?" I must hear that request a hundred times a day as a little outstretched arm holds up a brightly colored sippee cup. It makes me wonder if that is how God sees me sometimes, like a needy child constantly asking Him to please fill my cup. At times I thought maybe God had gotten a little distracted while pouring my portion and I felt like I was left soggy and stuck in the sticky overflow of blessings. Just as my kids sometimes scream, "I no yike dat kind," I, too, felt like stubbornly stomping my feet and yelling out to God, "I said one or two babies, not six!"

There was never a question in my mind of whether or not God loved me. It was just that sometimes I felt like a favorite childhood stuffed animal that had been loved to the point of being threadbare, limp, and lifeless. That's when I discovered a valuable aspect of God's love that I really hadn't tapped into before my endless hours as Mother to eight: mercy. Lamentations 3:22–23 says, "Because of the LORD's great love we are not consumed, for his compassions never fail. They are new every morning."

It was the "new every morning" part that wrapped itself around me like a great big hug. I realized that although God had certainly caused my "cup to runneth over," He loved me enough to give me a fresh start each and every day. That meant on those nights when I would lay my head on my pillow beating myself up over the fact that I had lost my patience with Mady during dinner, that I didn't take the time to clap as Alexis showed off her wobbly steps, or that I hadn't had the chance to sneak in a special hug for Joel that day, I could still rest in the reassurance that God's mercies are new every day. He loved me enough to see me through to the next morning where I had the chance once again to give it my best shot.

5. God will provide

Before the babies were born I would almost always have a pain in my stomach when I finally closed my checkbook after paying bills. One thing my father taught me was the importance of being financially responsible; but I found the pace at which money was deposited and then all too soon withdrawn from my bank account to be downright infuriating. I'd look with utter disgust at the stack of envelopes that looked like flat white hands held out to collect our hard-earned wages. "Why do I have to pay all of my money for this and this and this," I'd complain as I riffled through the pile. All of my financial stress was still at that time being fed by my childhood fear of not having enough.

And then came the babies.

My far-off fear suddenly became my very up-close reality. I didn't have enough — not enough arms, not enough room, not enough sleep, not enough time, not enough patience, not enough energy, and most assuredly, not enough money. Pushed to the brink of despair, I grabbed onto God's promise in Philippians 4:19 that says, "And my God will meet all your needs according to his glorious riches in Christ Jesus."

My needs were great, some as massive as the strength it would take to physically, mentally, and emotionally endure the actual birth of sextuplets; others were mundane and dull in comparison. For example, when the babies were very young, I kept a master list taped on the wall next to the mirror in the upstairs bathroom. We seemed to always need things like wipes, bottle liners, and even batteries for the bouncy seats — and because volunteers were always asking what they could bring, I hung my list where they washed their hands. One day on my way upstairs to jot paper towels on the list, I heard someone shuffling around outside the front door. Going to the door, I realized that one of my evening volunteers was wrestling with a large case of paper towels that someone had dropped off on our front steps. Pulling the cumbersome package inside, I just smiled to myself. By then I couldn't say I was surprised that God knew exactly what I needed even before it went on the list. I was just newly reminded that day that my God delivered.

Earlier in my life, I never could've imagined being thrilled and thankful over the gift of paper towels, but I had come a long way. I learned to be content with what I had, for there was a time when I truly didn't know what I was going to feed my girls for dinner. We had no money, food in my cabinets was sparse, plus I didn't even have the freedom to go get food. I was completely and utterly at the mercy of God and those He chose to put in my path. Under those circumstances, I found it ironic as I sat at the kitchen counter one day paying our monthly bills. I was no longer angry as the finished pile of envelopes stacked up beside me; instead, I was actually thankful. Each and every bill that I was able to pay only reminded me that God was providing for our family and miraculously seeing us through one day at a time.

6. Give God the glory and praise

I can't even count the number of times the phrase "Why me?" has gone through my head in the past three years. In the beginning, I would wonder why a God who was all-powerful and all-knowing could possibly think it was a good idea to give me six babies at one time. He didn't even design the human body to do that, and yet He had somehow touched *my* body, enabling it to stretch and conform to unnatural demands. In the midst of the pain, I'd ask, "But why me?"

Months later when I stood in the middle of my family room surrounded with wailing infants and their vast array of paraphernalia — pushed to my limits physically, emotionally, psychologically, and financially — I would look at my human weaknesses and limitations and continue to cry out, "Why me, Lord?" My world of absolutes had grown hazier and hazier and I felt lost, misguided, and forgotten.

Eventually though, as I slowly began to grow into my transformed life, I decided that I could either stay weighed down by that question, wearing it like a heavy worn out coat that hindered my mobility *or* I could choose to see it as carefully placed stepping stones put in my path to lead me closer to Him. Some of those stones were treacherously slippery, but it was at those times when I held on just a little tighter to the hand that never left my side.

With the clarity that hindsight often offers, I began to look back at the many opportunities Jon and I have had to tell about the miracles in our life, not only the actual birth of the babies but also the daily minute by minute sustenance that became a living witness to those around us. Although Jon and I desired to glorify God from the minute we committed to walk the long, arduous path He had laid out before us, it wasn't until the fog of the first two years lifted that I actually saw the answer to "Why me?" The answer lay not in what God had allowed to happen *to* us; instead it was what God hoped to accomplish *through* us.

I realized that our miraculous story of stubborn faith-driven persistence was being used by God, and had been used from the beginning, to bring glory and honor to Him. Even people who had initially scoffed at us could not deny the powerful testimony of love and grace. We observed the stunned awe in people's expressions when they saw our lineup of dark-haired toddlers bookended by Cara and Mady; and I have to say, I knew it made more than a few people stop in the busyness of their lives and acknowledge God's omnipotent power.

It was around that time that Jon and I were invited to speak at a large church. I knew it was an opportunity to allow God to be glorified through our lives, and yet I was distracted by the criticism that at times whirled around us. Feeling unworthy, I boldly dared to question God again. Did He really feel that I was the right person for the job, to stand up in front of people like I had everything under control? After all, I was known to be rather direct, blunt, and even dangerous with my mouth; and now God directed me to use the very thing that had always gotten me in so much trouble to instead bring glory to Him. I promptly reminded Him of all my faults and shortcomings, and He repeatedly reminded me that He was bigger.

I battled with my insecurities, and every time I'd lose my patience, I'd hear that nasty voice in my head saying I couldn't do it, that only people who exemplify goodness, grace, and gentleness can stand up in front of a crowd as an inspirational speaker. That's when I had an epiphany: possibly for the first time in my life, I realized that it was exactly because I *wasn't* perfect that God was willing to use me.

Today I stand in my kitchen with six three-year-olds lined up at the large window in the living room waving jubilantly at Mady and Cara as they step off the school bus at the end of the driveway. It's already been a very long day; three of the kids have had a winter bug, we're in the middle of getting new carpet installed upstairs, and our Big Blue Bus wouldn't start this morning. Nevertheless I look at them dancing around excitedly as the girls come in to greet them and I can hardly believe this is my life.

I feel so incredibly blessed that God has chosen us for this journey. This life is absolutely not in a million years what Jon and I expected, but it is infinitely more than we ever hoped or dreamed in so many ways. While Jon and I can't imagine what the days ahead will hold for our family, I am often comforted by a quote by Abraham Lincoln. He said, "The best thing about the future is that it comes one day at a time." I say, "Thank God."

Kate's Journal

● ● ● ● ●

I'm still here !!!! My ~~feel~~ feeling
is that I'll last to 30wks ∞

∞ and not too much beyond --just
my gut feeling. But if God gives
me the endurance and strength,
I'll go as far as He wants me
to go! I love our 6 babies and
I want them to do well so I will
suffer, even though I feel very
selfish a lot lately & want this
~~over with~~! I am sooooo miserable!
And that is an understatement!
Here's my complaint list:
    1) my belly goes ~ 4 inches shy
    of to my knees when I sit.
    It is so heavy & hurts. I can't
    sit or stand long. It's hard to
    walk now & showering is next
    to impossible.

Like a bad sunburn! → 2) The cervix on my lower right
    side of my belly is so sore

3) US are pure torture. I can't breathe + it kills my back
4) I pee constantly at night

and the ridiculous residents wake me up @ the crack of dawn for stupidity !!!!
5) my back (lower) hurts sooooo bad
6) I contract constantly + they hurt and are annoying!
Anyway, Tuesday was the next growth scans. Here are their latest weights:

(gained 9oz) Baby A: 2LB 11OZ
? Baby B: 2 LB 5oz ? measurement
(gained 3oz) Baby C: 2LB 3oz
(gained 7oz) Baby D: 2LB 10oz
(gained 5oz) Baby E: 2LB 14oz
(gained 4oz) Baby F: 2LB 14oz
                          _____
                          15LB 9oz

Acknowledgments

Thank you again, anyone and everyone, including nurses, doctors, volunteers, individuals, friends, family, strangers, companies, businesses, churches, and neighbors who have had any part in helping our family along the way during our ever changing journey. We know that each of you played an important part and nothing big or small has gone unnoticed or unappreciated!

Jon & Kate's Photo Album

• • • • •

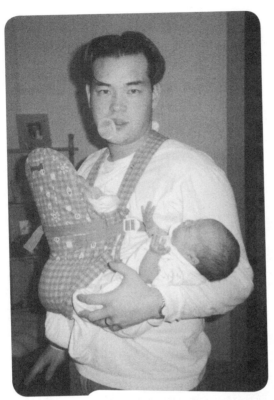

Super Dad

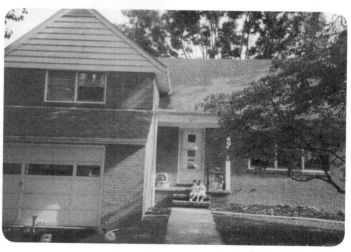

Our first house. We were so proud of it!

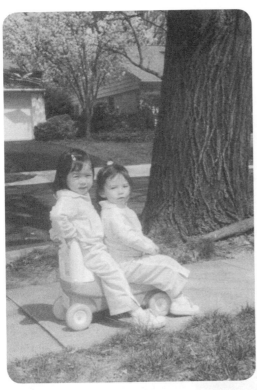

Cara and Mady around the time that we had the chance to adopt, May 2003.

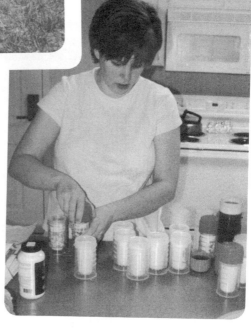

Settling into a bottle making routine in our condo.

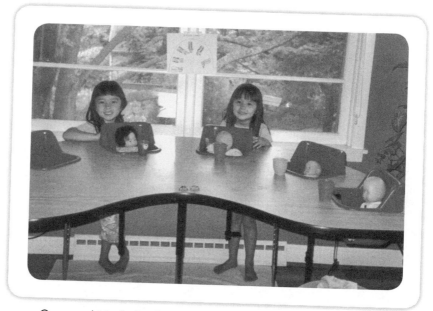

Cara and Mady feeding their babies in between real feedings.

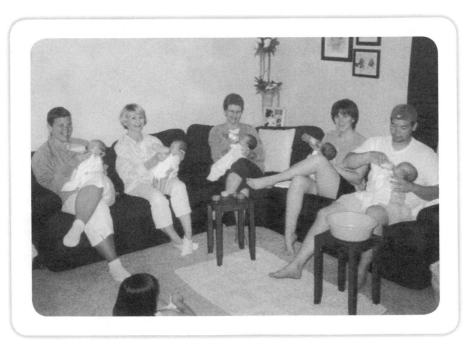

Five of six baby feeders.

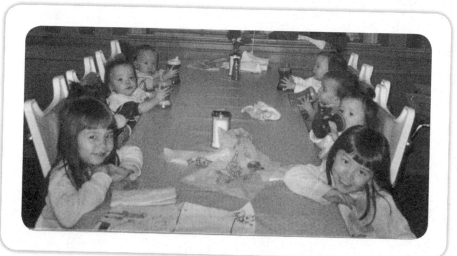

Out to dinner as a family for the first time.

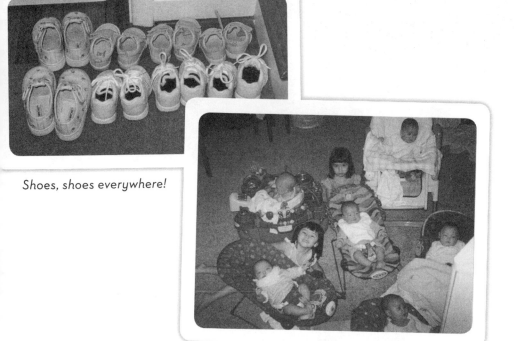

Shoes, shoes everywhere!

A typical sight at five months. Clockwise: Cara, Leah (in high chair), Alexis, Hannah, Joel, Mady, Aaden, and Collin in center.

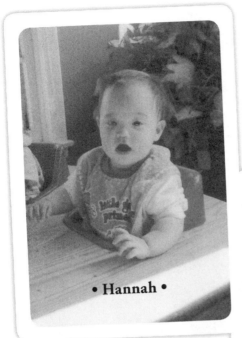

• Hannah •

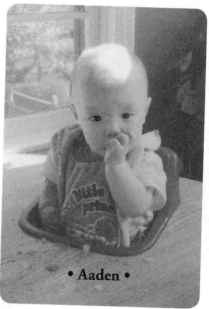

• Aaden •

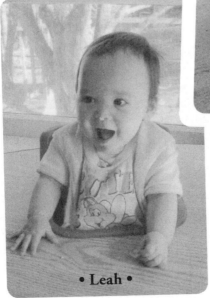

• Leah •

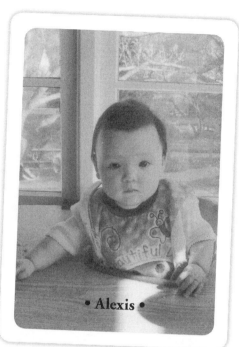

• Alexis •

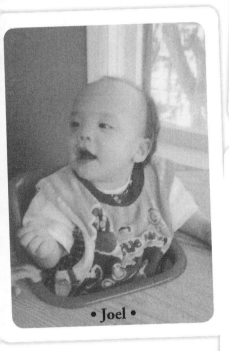

• Joel •

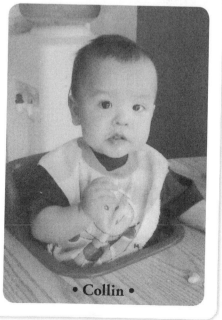

• Collin •

For recent information, stories,
and updates on our family, please visit
www.sixgosselins.com.

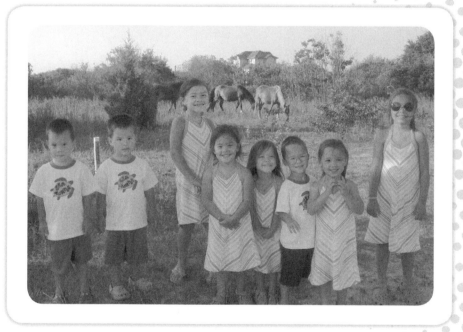

Share Your Thoughts

With the Author: Your comments will be forwarded to the author when you send them to *zauthor@zondervan.com*.

With Zondervan: Submit your review of this book by writing to *zreview@zondervan.com*.

Free Online Resources at
www.zondervan.com/hello

 Zondervan AuthorTracker: Be notified whenever your favorite authors publish new books, go on tour, or post an update about what's happening in their lives.

 Daily Bible Verses and Devotions: Enrich your life with daily Bible verses or devotions that help you start every morning focused on God.

 Free Email Publications: Sign up for newsletters on fiction, Christian living, church ministry, parenting, and more.

 Zondervan Bible Search: Find and compare Bible passages in a variety of translations at www.zondervanbiblesearch.com.

 Other Benefits: Register yourself to receive online benefits like coupons and special offers, or to participate in research.

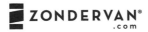